LECTIN FREE SNACKS

COOKBOOK

Fight inflammation with easy to follow food list and dessert recipes to achieve optimum gut health.

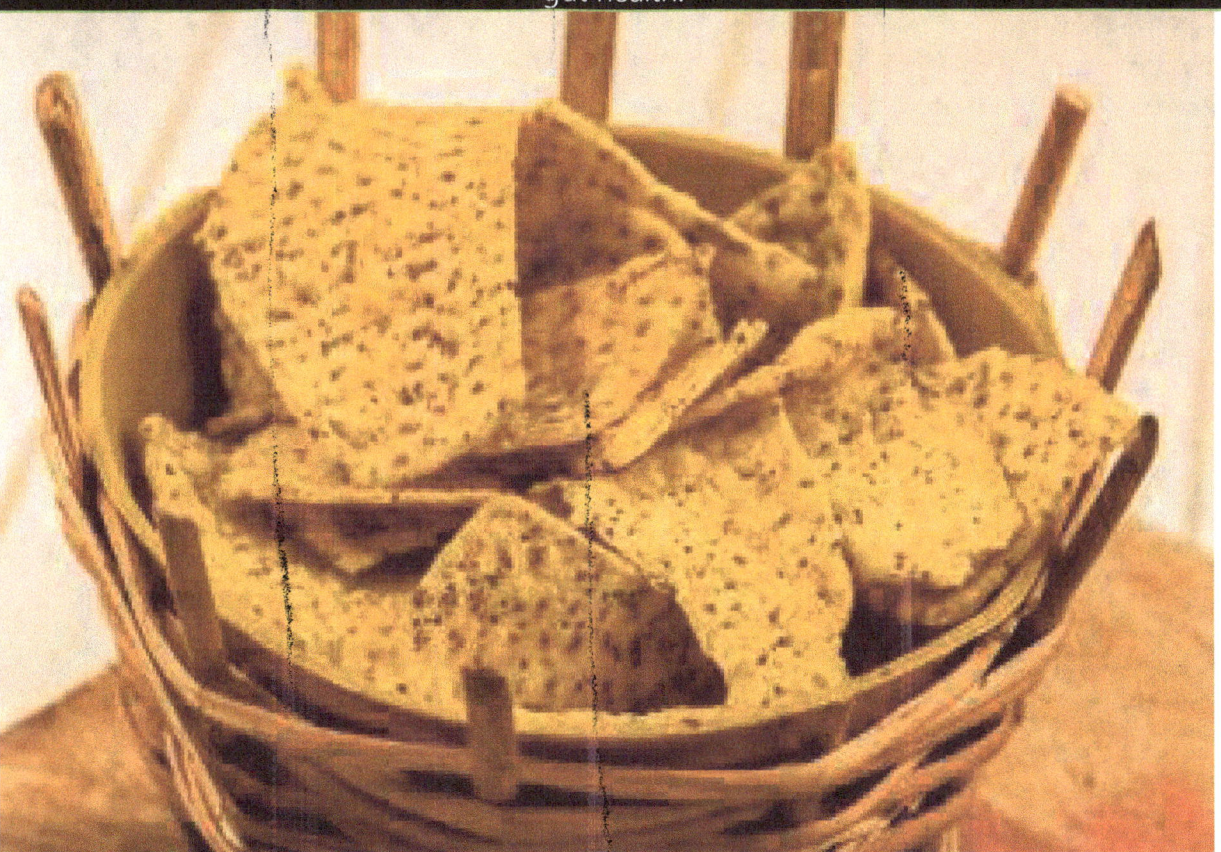

Angela Rachel Staten

Copyright Page

Copyright ©2024 by Angela Rachel Staten

All rights reserved. No part of this book may be reproduced or transmitted in any form or by any means, electronic or mechanical, including photocopying, recording, or by any information storage and retrieval system, without permission in writing from the publisher

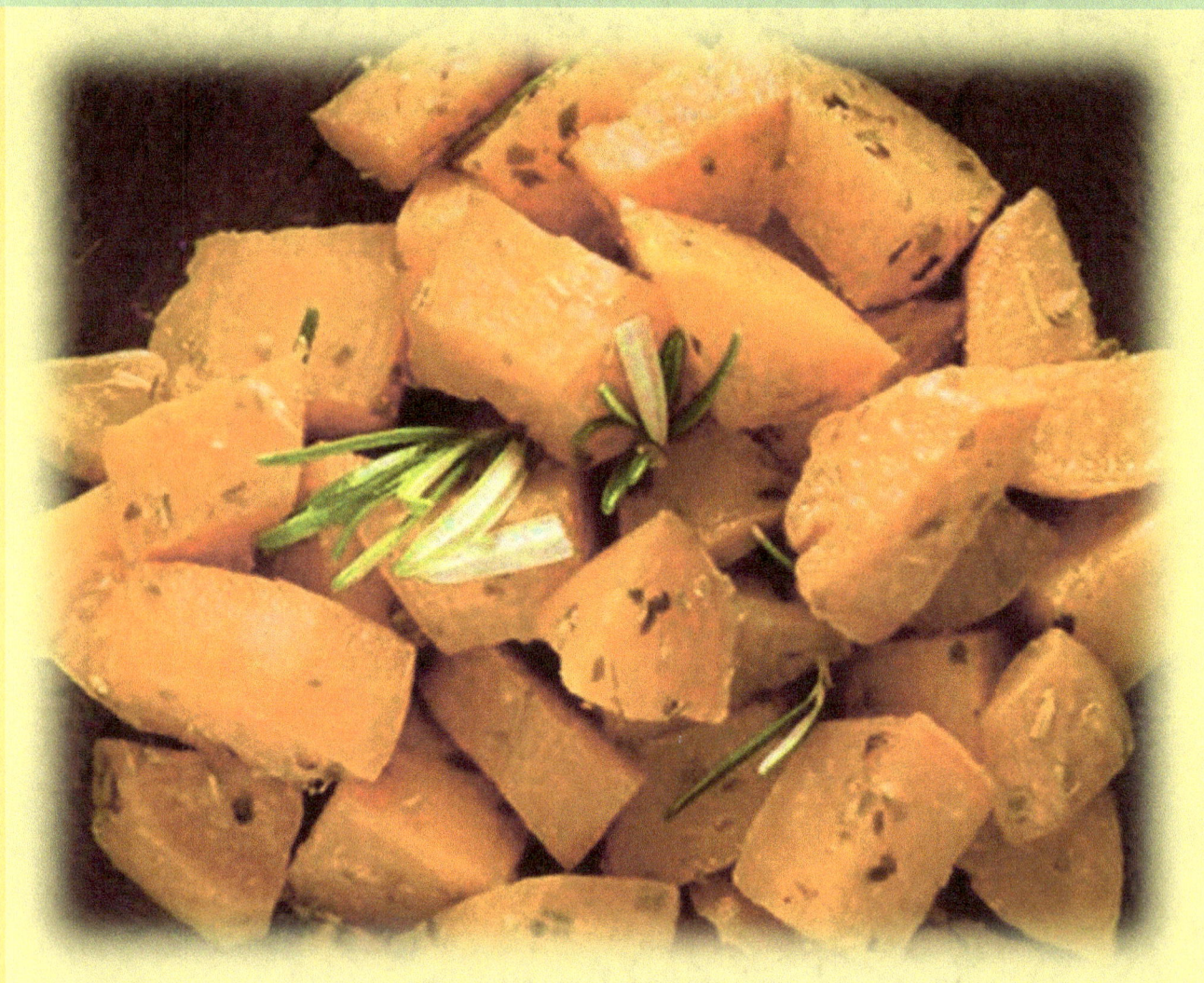

Disclaimer: The recipes contained in this cookbook are intended for personal use and enjoyment. The author and publisher are not responsible for any health issues or allergic reactions that may arise from the use of the ingredients or recipes provided. It is recommended that individuals with specific dietary concerns or restrictions consult a qualified healthcare professional.

ABOUT THE AUTHOR

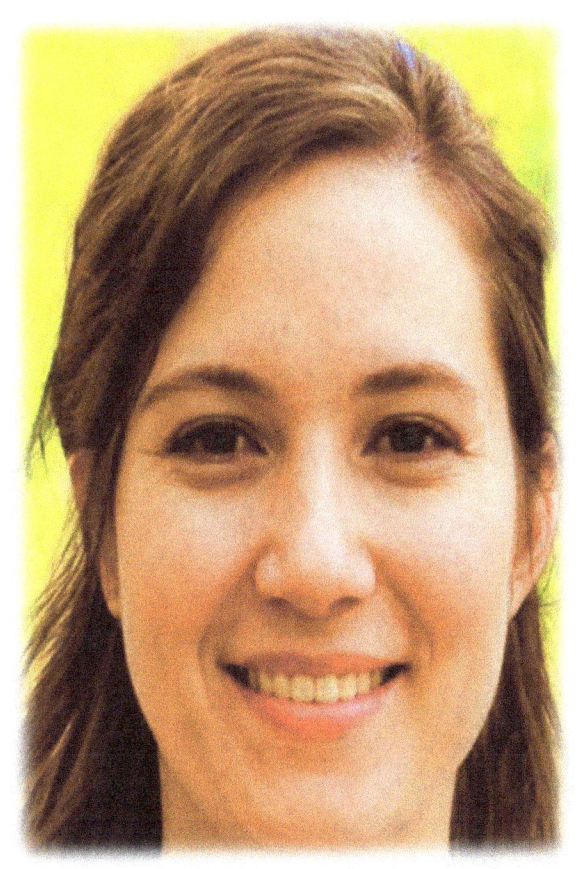

Whether you have osteoarthritis or are facing another health issue, my intention is not to give you a ton of confusing guidelines.

Rather, I wish to provide you with the means to effect long-term change.

One of the greatest methods to achieve this is by following a healthy diet, which focuses on eating tasty but simple foods that will fuel your body and provide you with the strongest defense against illness.

My name is Angela Rachel Staten, and I'm a medical professional and qualified nutritionist who is totally committed to using food as medicine.

Although it may sound generic, I have personally witnessed the profound impact that a healthy diet can have on people's lives. I am a case study in action.

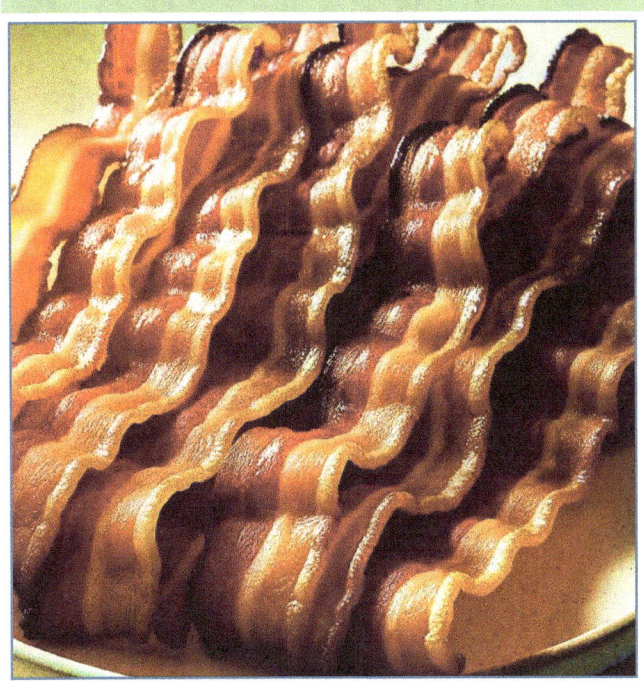

What you will find in this book:

- Clear explanations of the nutritional value of food and how it affects leading a healthy lifestyle.

- Scrumptious meals that genuinely inspire a desire for healthy eating.

- Some pointers for incorporating this diet into your busy lifestyle.

- Consider myself your companion in this. One delectable, nutritious meal at a time, I'm here to help you on your path to feeling better.

So unwind and let's get started.

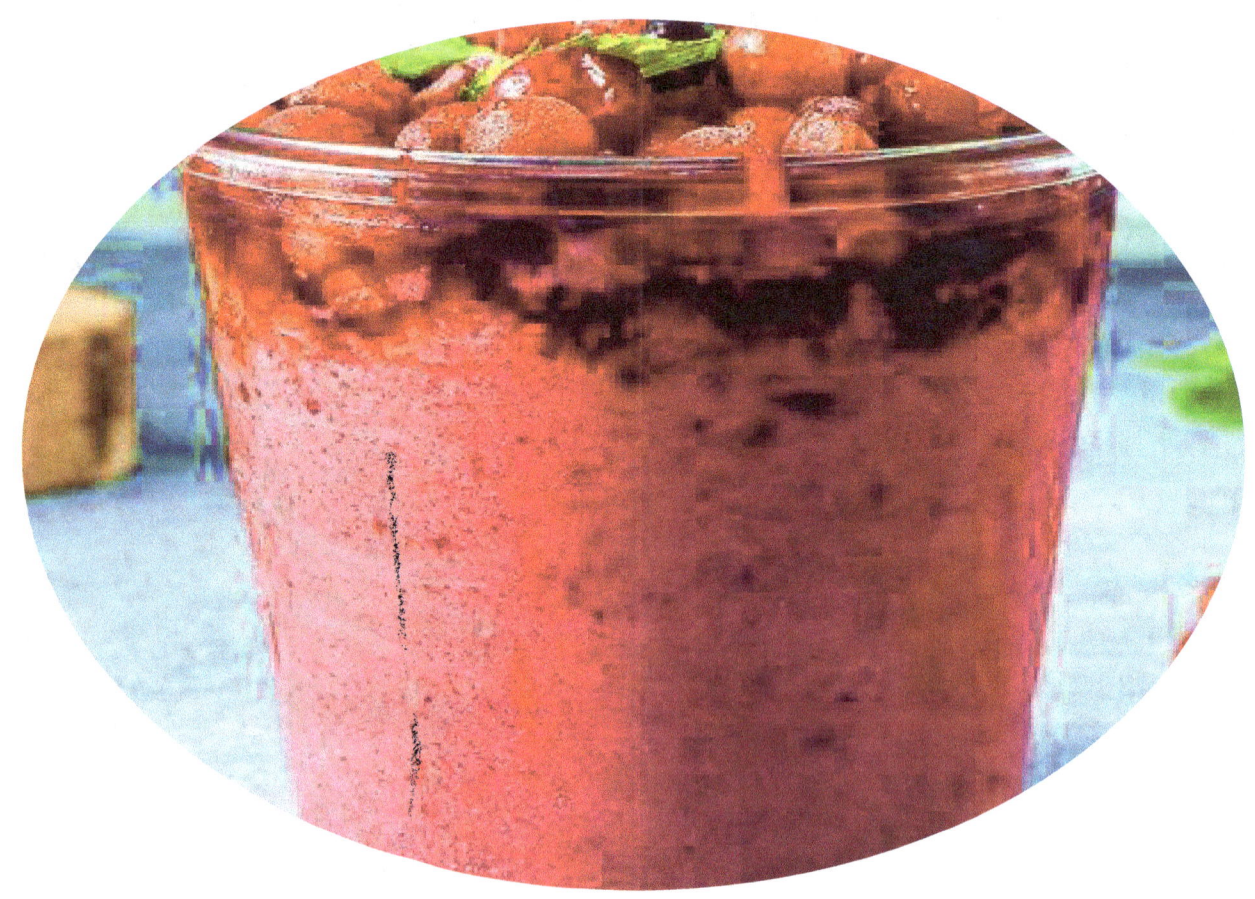

UNIQUE TABLE OF CONTENT

What you will find in this book: 4
INTRODUCTION 9
Understanding Lectins and Their Impact on Health 11
   Potential Benefits of Lectins: 11
   Potential Concerns of Lectins: 11
Benefits of Adopting a Lectin-Free Diet 12
   Proponents of the diet believe it can offer various health benefits, including: 12
   Important Considerations: 12
   Here's what you'll find inside: 13
BASICS OF LECTIN FREE SNACKING 15
   Structure and Types of Lectins: 16
   Lectins and Digestion: 16
   Individual Sensitivity to Lectins: 17
   What Are Lectin-Free Snacks? 17
Basic Cooking Tools: 20
   Cooking Techniques: 20
BREAKFAST 23
RECIPES 23
. Spicy Trail Mix 24
Creamy Avocado Dip with Carrot Sticks 25
Berry Bliss Smoothie 26
Herb-Roasted Almonds 27
Zesty Cucumber Salad with Chia Seeds 28

Apple Nachos with Cinnamon-Coconut Drizzle 29
Mini Frittata Cups with Broccoli and Cheddar 30
No-Bake Energy Bites with Dates and Walnuts 31
Tropical Fruit Skewers with Lime and Mint 32
Simple Green Salad with Lemon Vinaigrette 33
Nutrient-Packed Lectin-Free Snacks for Energy 35
Power Veggie Sticks with Creamy Avocado Dip 36
Berry Bliss Smoothie Bowl 37
Spiced Nut & Seed Trail Mix 38
Crispy Coconut Chips with Citrus Dip 39
Zucchini Noodle Primavera 40
Apple Slices with Almond Butter 41
Frittata Bites with Fresh Herbs 42
Pear and Pecan Energy Balls 43
Pumpkin Seed & Celery Seed Hummus 44
Spiced Melon Skewers with Coconut Yogurt Dip 45
Creative Lectin-Free Snacks for Every Occasion 47
Elegant Caprese Skewers with Balsamic Glaze 48
Mini Bell Pepper Poppers Stuffed with Cashew Cheese 49
Festive Guacamole Cups with Plantain Chips 50
Savory Mushroom and Spinach Pinwheels for Party Platters ... 51
Decadent Desserts Sans Lectins 53
Spiced Berry Crumble with Coconut Topping 54
Creamy Avocado Mousse with Citrus Glaze 55
Tropical Fruit Salad with Toasted Nut and Seed Crunch 56

Decadent Paleo Chocolate Bars 57

Refreshing Mint and Melon Sorbet 58

Spiced Pear and Almond Butter Fritters 59

Coconut and Pecan Cookies with a Hint of Cinnamon 60

Kid-Friendly Lectin-Free Snack Creations 61

Ant on a Log 63

Rainbow Veggie Sticks with Dip 64

Mini "Pizzas" on Sliced Apples 65

Sweet & Savory Trail Mix 66

Frozen Yogurt Bites 67

Spiced Coconut Crackers 68

Gluten-Free and Lectin-Free Options 69

Spicy Shrimp and Veggie Stir-Fry 70

Coconut Curried Chicken Salad 71

Zucchini Noodle Primavera 72

Almond Flour Pancakes 73

Baked Salmon with Herb Crust (Gluten-Free & Lectin-Free) ... 74

Dairy-Free and Lectin-Free Substitutions 75

Creamy Avocado Pasta Sauce 76

Coconut Yogurt Parfait 77

Cauliflower Rice Soup 78

Avocado Toast with Poached Eggs 79

Tropical Smoothie Bowl 80

Vegan and Lectin-Free Recipes for Plant-Based Enthusiasts ... 81

Lentil Soup with Vegetables 82

Black Bean Burgers..83
Tofu Scramble 84
Roasted Chickpea Salad with Herbs.......................................85
Vegan Lectin-Free Coconut Curry with Vegetables................86
Conclusion 88

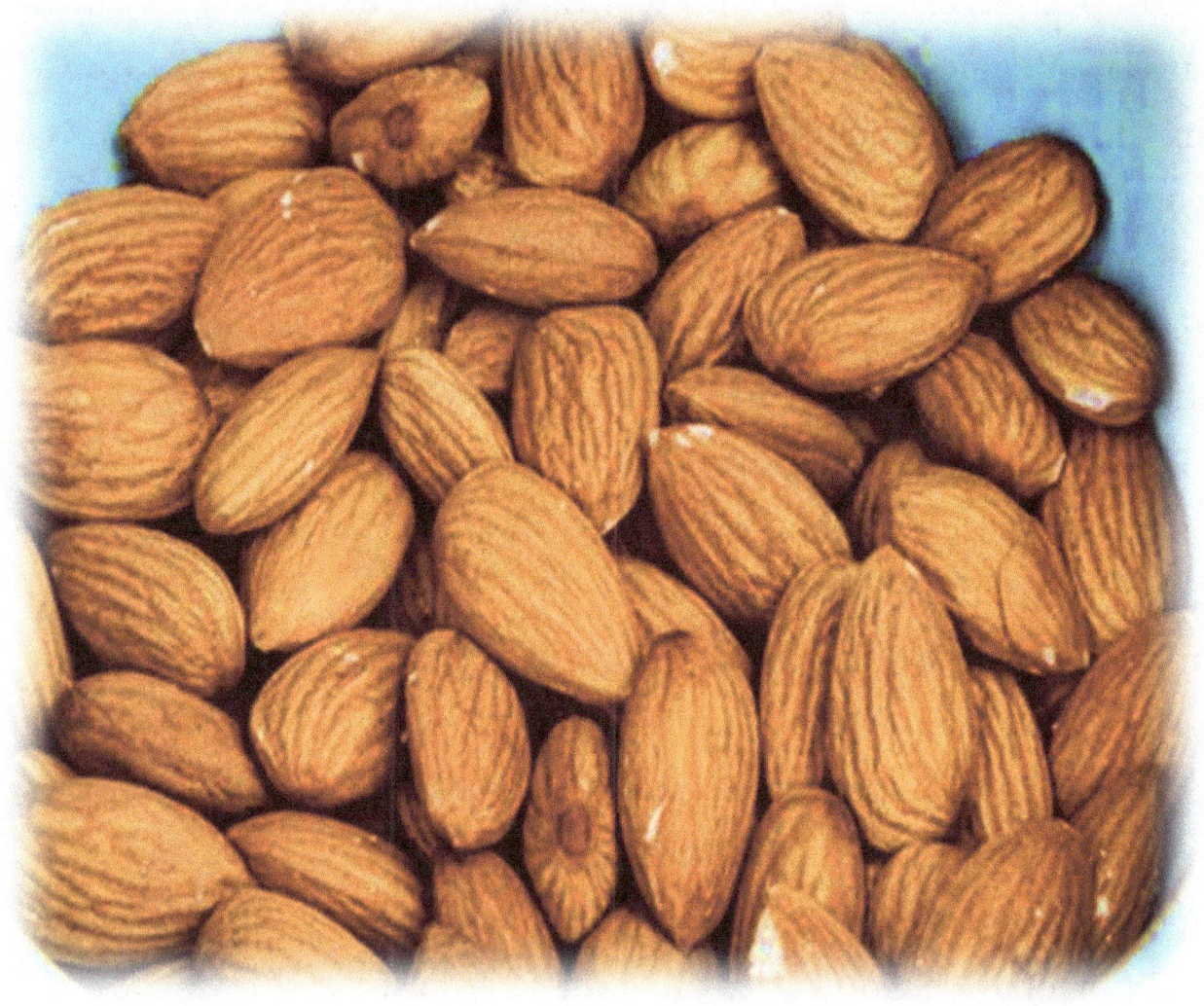

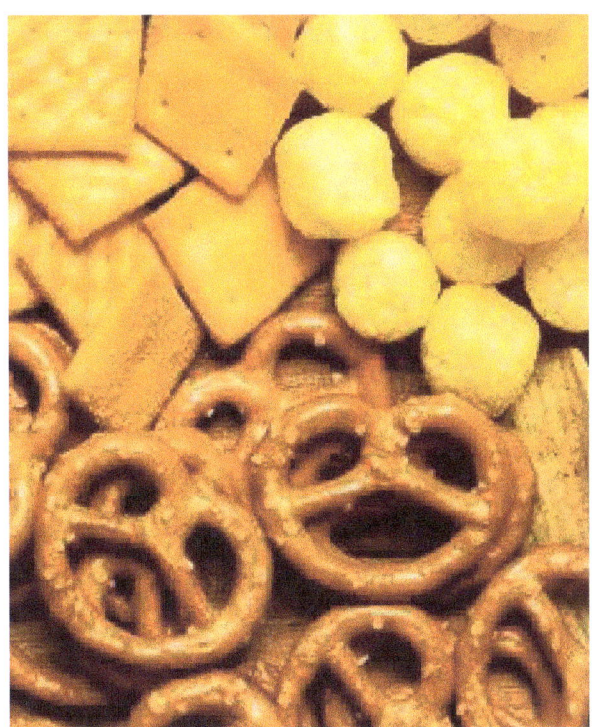

INTRODUCTION

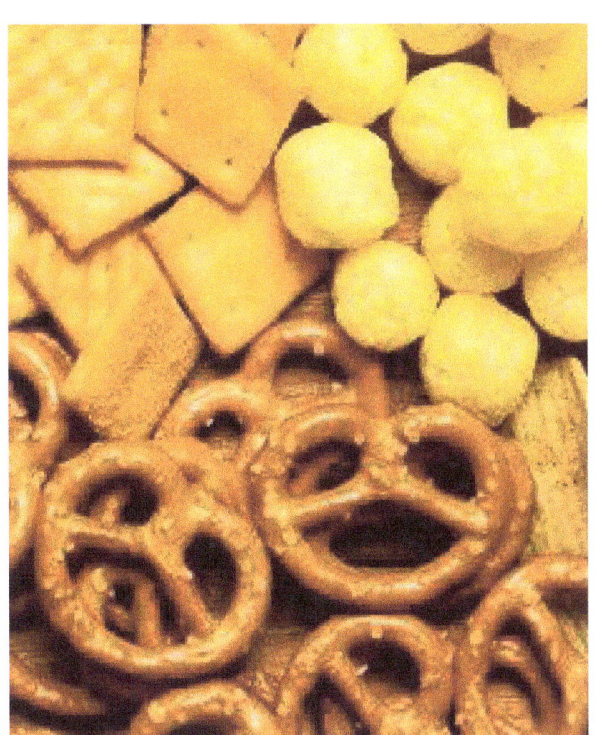

Ever dreamed of ditching the guilt and indulging in delicious snacks that nourish your body? Welcome to the wonderful world of lectin-free treats! This book is your passport to a vibrant snacking adventure, one free from bloating and full of flavor.

Forget bland and boring! We'll unlock a treasure trove of sweet and savory delights, from bite-sized protein powerhouses to portable snacks that fuel your day. Dive into creamy dips and refreshing crudités for effortless entertaining, or whip up decadent desserts that redefine indulgence.

Whether you're a seasoned lectin-free pro or just embarking on this journey, this book is your one-stop shop for healthy, satisfying snacks. Let's transform your snacking routine and show you how lectin-free living can be anything but restrictive. It's time to unleash your inner snacking genius – lectin-free style!

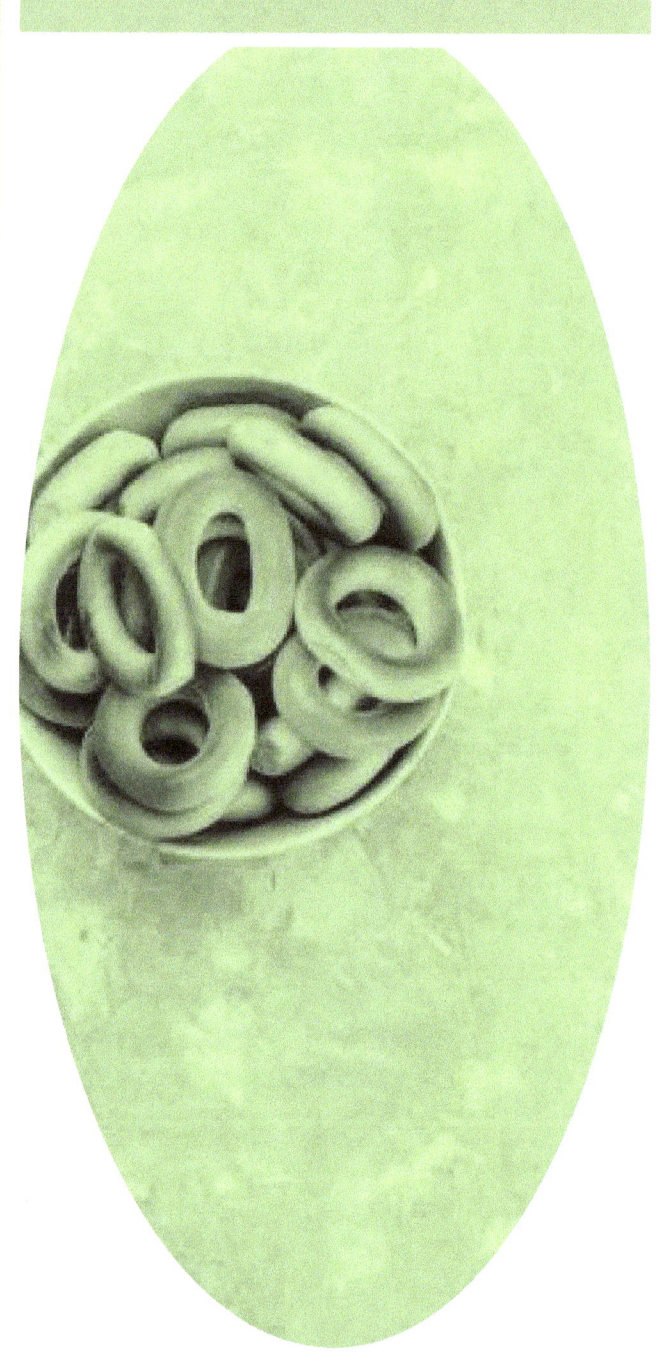

Understanding Lectins and Their Impact on Health

Lectins are a group of proteins naturally found in various plants, including legumes (beans, lentils, peanuts), grains (wheat, barley, rye), some vegetables (nightshades like tomatoes, potatoes, and peppers), and even some fruits. While lectins play a role in the plant's defense system against predators, their impact on human health remains a topic of ongoing research and debate.

Potential Benefits of Lectins:

Plant Defense: Lectins can bind to carbohydrates on the surface of insect and fungal cells, potentially aiding the plant in warding off these threats.

Nutrient Binding: Some lectins may help plants retain essential minerals like manganese and magnesium.

Potential Concerns of Lectins:

Digestive Discomfort: Lectins are resistant to human digestion. They can bind to the lining of the gut, potentially leading to digestive issues like bloating, gas, and diarrhea in some individuals, particularly those with sensitive digestive systems.

Leaky Gut Syndrome: Some theories propose that lectins might contribute to leaky gut syndrome, a condition where the gut lining becomes more permeable, allowing the passage of unwanted substances into the bloodstream. To validate this connection, more investigation is necessary.

Autoimmune Issues: There's limited evidence suggesting lectins might mimic certain sugars found on human cells, potentially triggering an autoimmune response in susceptible individuals.

It's important to note:

The lectin content in foods can vary depending on factors like the specific plant variety, growing conditions, and preparation methods.

Cooking methods like soaking, sprouting, boiling, and pressure cooking can significantly reduce lectin content.

Not everyone experiences negative effects from lectins. Many people consume lectin-containing foods without any issues.

Benefits of Adopting a Lectin-Free Diet

Proponents of the diet believe it can offer various health benefits, including:

Improved Digestion: By removing lectins that may irritate the gut lining, the lectin-free diet may lead to reduced bloating, gas, and other digestive discomforts.

Decreased Inflammation: Chronic inflammation has been connected to a number of health issues. Some studies suggest lectins might contribute to inflammation. A lectin-free diet may help lessen inflammation, potentially improving overall health.

Weight Management: Lectin-free foods tend to be higher in protein and fiber, promoting satiety and potentially aiding in weight management efforts.

Enhanced Energy Levels: Digestive issues and inflammation can drain energy levels. By addressing these concerns, a lectin-free diet could lead to increased energy and vitality.

Improved Skin Health: Some believe lectins may contribute to skin problems like acne and eczema. Eliminating them could potentially improve skin health.

Important Considerations:

The lectin-free diet is a relatively new concept with limited scientific research to support its long-term health benefits.

Restrictive diets can be challenging to maintain and may lead to nutritional deficiencies if not carefully planned. Consulting a registered dietitian is crucial to ensure you're getting all the essential nutrients while following a lectin-free approach.

The lectin-free diet may not be suitable for everyone. It's best to discuss it with your doctor before making significant dietary changes.

How This Cookbook Can Help You Enjoy Delicious Snacks Without Lectins

Going lectin-free doesn't mean sacrificing flavor or variety when it comes to snacking. This cookbook is your guide to creating a delicious and satisfying snack repertoire that aligns with the lectin-free philosophy.

Here's what you'll find inside:

A Wide Range of Recipes: From savory protein-packed bites to refreshing sweet treats, this book offers a plethora of snack ideas to satisfy different cravings.

Focus on Fresh, Whole Foods: The recipes prioritize fresh, wholesome ingredients with naturally low lectin content. You'll discover a world of vibrant vegetables, nuts, seeds, and delicious fruits.

Easy and Accessible Recipes: The recipes are designed to be easy to follow, with clear instructions and readily available ingredients. You won't need any hard-to-find specialty items to create these delicious snacks.

Dietary Modifications: Many recipes offer suggestions for substitutions to cater to specific dietary needs or preferences.

Meal Planning Tips: The book provides guidance on planning your lectin-free snacks and incorporating them into your daily routine.

By using this cookbook, you can:

Break Free from Bland Snacks: Ditch the processed, sugary snacks and discover exciting new lectin-free options that tantalize your taste buds.

Fuel Your Body with Goodness: These snacks are packed with essential nutrients to keep

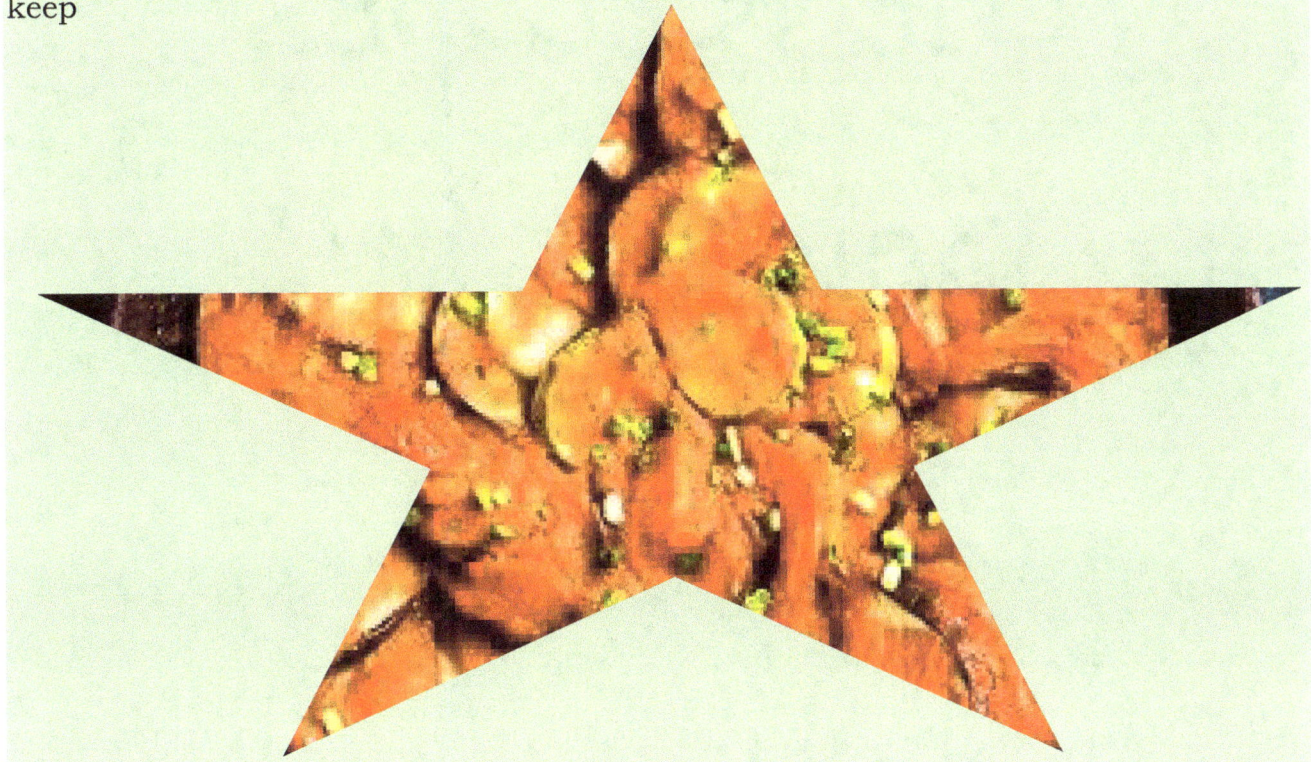

"The Right Snacks can Aid Longevity since the Recipes Don't Lie"

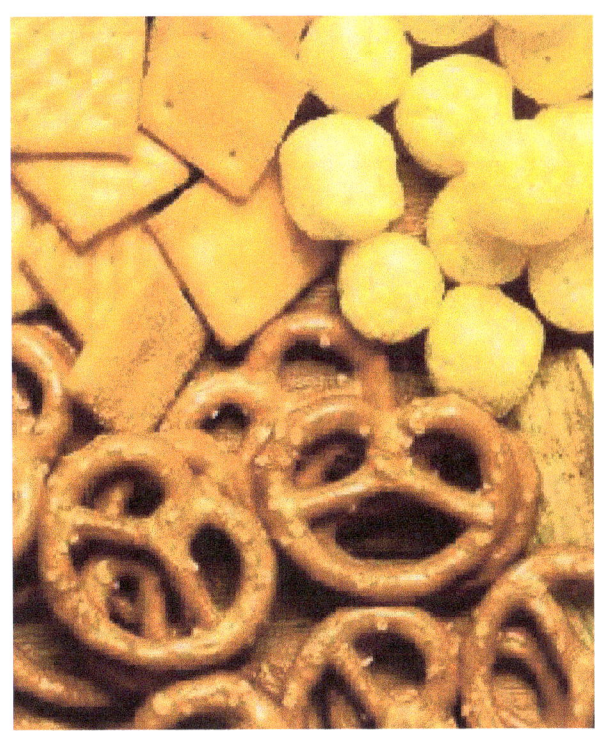

BASICS OF LECTIN FREE SNACKING

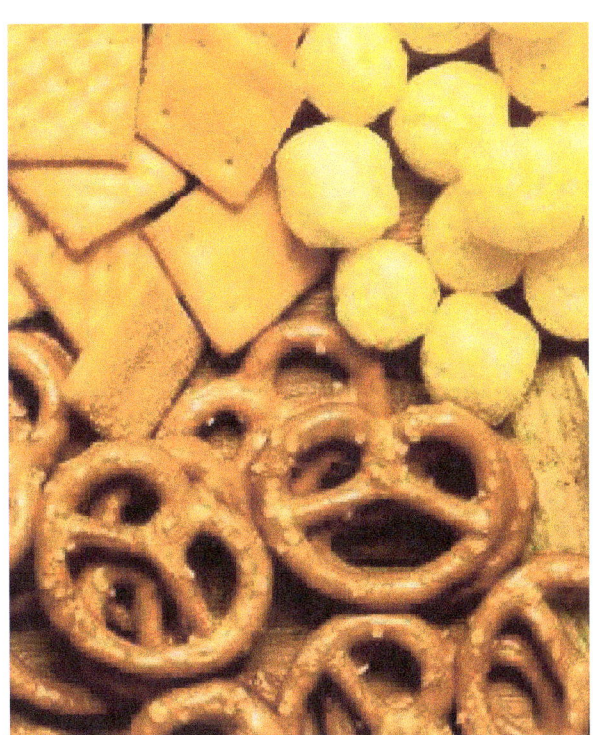

Delving Deeper into Lectins: Friends or Foes?

Lectins are a complex group of proteins naturally found in various plants. They play a crucial role in the plant's defense system, binding to sugars on the surface of insects and fungi, potentially inhibiting their growth or causing them harm. While lectins offer the plant a survival advantage, their impact on human health remains a topic of ongoing research and debate.

Structure and Types of Lectins:

Lectins have a specific structure that allows them to bind to carbohydrates. This binding ability can have consequences for human digestion depending on the type of lectin and the individual's sensitivity. There are numerous lectin types, with some of the most common ones found in:

Legumes: Beans, lentils, peanuts (although peanuts are technically legumes, they are often classified separately due to their unique properties)

Grains: Wheat, barley, rye

Nightshade Vegetables: Tomatoes, potatoes, peppers, eggplant

Certain Fruits: Squash, melons

Lectins and Digestion:

The human digestive system lacks the specific enzymes needed to completely break down lectins. Several possible problems may result from this:

Gut Irritation: Undigested lectins can bind to the lining of the gut, causing irritation and discomfort. This can manifest as bloating, gas, diarrhea, and abdominal pain in some individuals.

Leaky Gut Syndrome: Some theories suggest lectins might contribute to leaky gut syndrome, a condition where the gut lining becomes more permeable, allowing the passage of unwanted substances into the bloodstream. While research is ongoing, a leaky gut is linked to various health problems.

Autoimmune Concerns: Limited evidence suggests lectins might mimic certain sugars found on human cells, potentially triggering an autoimmune response in susceptible individuals. However, more research is required to solidify this link.

It's important to note:

The lectin content in foods can vary depending on several factors, including:

Plant Variety: Different varieties within the same plant family might have varying lectin levels.

Growing Conditions: Factors like soil quality and sun exposure could influence lectin content.

Preparation Methods: Certain cooking methods like soaking, sprouting, boiling, and pressure cooking can significantly reduce lectin content.

Individual Sensitivity to Lectins:

Not everyone experiences negative effects from lectins. Many people consume lectin-containing foods without any issues. However, those with pre-existing gut problems or sensitivities might be more prone to experiencing discomfort.

What Are Lectin-Free Snacks?

Lectin-free snacks are essentially snacks that prioritize ingredients with minimal or no lectin content. Following a lectin-free approach to snacking can offer several potential benefits:

Improved Gut Health: By eliminating lectins that may irritate the gut lining, lectin-free snacks could lead to reduced digestive discomforts.

Enhanced Energy Levels: Digestive issues and inflammation can drain energy levels. By potentially addressing these concerns, lectin-free snacks could lead to increased energy and vitality.

Overall Well-being: Proponents of the lectin-free diet believe it can contribute to improved overall well-being by addressing potential inflammation and gut issues.

Here's what makes a snack lectin-free:

Focus on Fresh, Whole Foods: Fruits, vegetables (excluding nightshades), nuts, and seeds are generally considered lectin-free or have very low lectin content.

Limited Grains and Legumes: Since most grains and legumes contain lectins, lectin-free snacks typically avoid them or use lectin-reduced options like sprouted grains.

Nightshade Exclusion (Optional): While not everyone reacts poorly to nightshade vegetables, some individuals choose to eliminate them for additional gut health benefits. This cookbook will offer recipes with and without nightshade options.–

Remember:

The lectin-free diet is a relatively new concept with limited long-term research.

Seeking advice from a certified dietitian is imperative to guarantee that, while adhering to a lectin-free diet, you are receiving all the necessary nutrients.

Not everybody can follow a lectin-free diet. It's best to discuss it with your doctor before making significant dietary changes.

This cookbook empowers you to create delicious and healthy lectin-free snacks. With a focus on whole foods and creative recipes, you can enjoy a variety of snacks that are both satisfying and potentially beneficial for your gut health and overall well-being.

Lectin-Free Pantry Essentials: Fueling Your Delicious Snacking Adventure

Going lectin-free doesn't mean sacrificing flavor or variety in your pantry. Here's a breakdown of key ingredients to keep on hand for creating a world of delicious lectin-free snacks:

Fresh Produce:

Vegetables (excluding nightshades): bell peppers (optional, if tolerated), carrots, celery, cucumbers, zucchini, mushrooms, asparagus, broccoli, cauliflower, and leafy greens (kale, spinach). These supply vital nutrients, vitamins, and fiber.

Fruits: berries (strawberries, blueberries, raspberries), apples, pears, oranges, grapefruit, kiwi, and melons (cantaloupe, honeydew). Lectin content in fruits is generally low, and they offer a natural sweetness for snacks. Optional: If tolerated, include bananas and grapes.

Fresh herbs: basil, cilantro, parsley, rosemary, and thyme. These add vibrant flavor to dips, salads, and cooked snacks.

Nuts and seeds:

Almonds are an excellent source of fiber, protein, and good fats. Enjoy them raw, roasted, or slivered for salads and trail mixes.

Walnuts: Rich in Omega-3 fatty acids, antioxidants, and fiber. Use them chopped in dips, spreads, or baked goods.

Pecans: Add a buttery flavor to snacks. Enjoy them whole, chopped, or candied (use lectin-free sweetener if making them yourself).

Pumpkin Seeds (Pepitas): A good source of protein, healthy fats, and zinc. Enjoy them raw, roasted, or ground into nut butter alternatives.–

Chia seeds have a lot of omega-3 fatty acids and fiber. They can be soaked in liquids to create a gel-like texture for puddings and parfaits.

Flax seeds are another great source of fiber and omega-3 fatty acids. Grind them fresh for maximum nutritional benefit, and use them in baked goods or sprinkled on snacks. Optional: Hemp seeds (if tolerated) offer a similar nutritional profile.

Healthy Fats:

Avocado is a creamy, nutrient-dense fruit rich in healthy fats and fiber. Perfect for guacamole, dips, or simply mashed on its own.

Coconut Oil: A versatile oil with a mild coconut flavor. Use it for cooking, baking, or as a base for homemade salad dressings.

Extra Virgin Olive Oil: A staple for most kitchens. Use it for drizzling, dressing, or light sautéing.

Other Pantry Staples:

Apple Cider Vinegar: Adds a tangy flavor to dips, dressings, and marinades.

Sea salt is essential for seasoning and can be used in various grinds.

Black pepper is a classic spice that adds warmth and depth of flavor.

Spices: Experiment with different spices to create flavor profiles for various snacks, such as cumin, turmeric, paprika, chili powder (optional, if nightshade avoiders tolerate it), and cinnamon.

Coconut Flour or Almond Flour: Great alternatives to wheat flour for baking lectin-free treats. They are high in fiber and add a unique texture. Optional: Arrowroot flour (if tolerated) can be used as a thickener.

Additional Considerations:

Dried Fruits: While technically lectin-free, be mindful of added sugars in some commercially available dried fruits. Choose unsweetened varieties whenever possible.

Lectin-Free Sweeteners: Explore options like stevia, erythritol, or monk fruit to add sweetness to snacks without the lectins found in sugar.–

Basic Cooking Tools:

Sharp Knives: A good chef's knife and a paring knife are essential for chopping, slicing, and dicing your ingredients.

Cutting Board: Choose a sturdy cutting board to protect your countertops and fingers.

Mixing Bowls: A variety of sizes will help you prepare different components of your snacks.

Measuring Cups and Spoons: Ensure accurate measurements for successful recipe execution.

Sheet pan: perfect for roasting vegetables, nuts, and seeds, or baking homemade crackers and chips.

Baking Dish: Useful for creating baked snacks like frittatas, energy bites, or muffins.

Food Processor (Optional): While not essential, a food processor can make tasks like chopping nuts, shredding vegetables, or making dips and spreads easier and faster.

Blender (optional): Great for creating smooth dips, sauces, and nut butter alternatives.

Lectin-Free Specific Tools (Optional):

(Optional): A spiralizer can transform vegetables like zucchini and sweet potatoes into fun noodles for a creative snack option

Cooking Techniques:

Roasting: Roasting vegetables, nuts, and seeds brings out their natural sweetness and deepens their flavor.

Sautéing is great for quickly cooking vegetables or creating flavorful bases for dips and sauces.

Baking: From savory frittatas to sweet cookies, baking allows you to create a variety of lectin-free snacks.

Chopping and Slicing: Mastering knife skills allows you to prepare fresh ingredients efficiently and create visually appealing snacks.

Blending and Processing: These techniques help achieve smooth textures in dips, sauces, and nut butter alternatives.

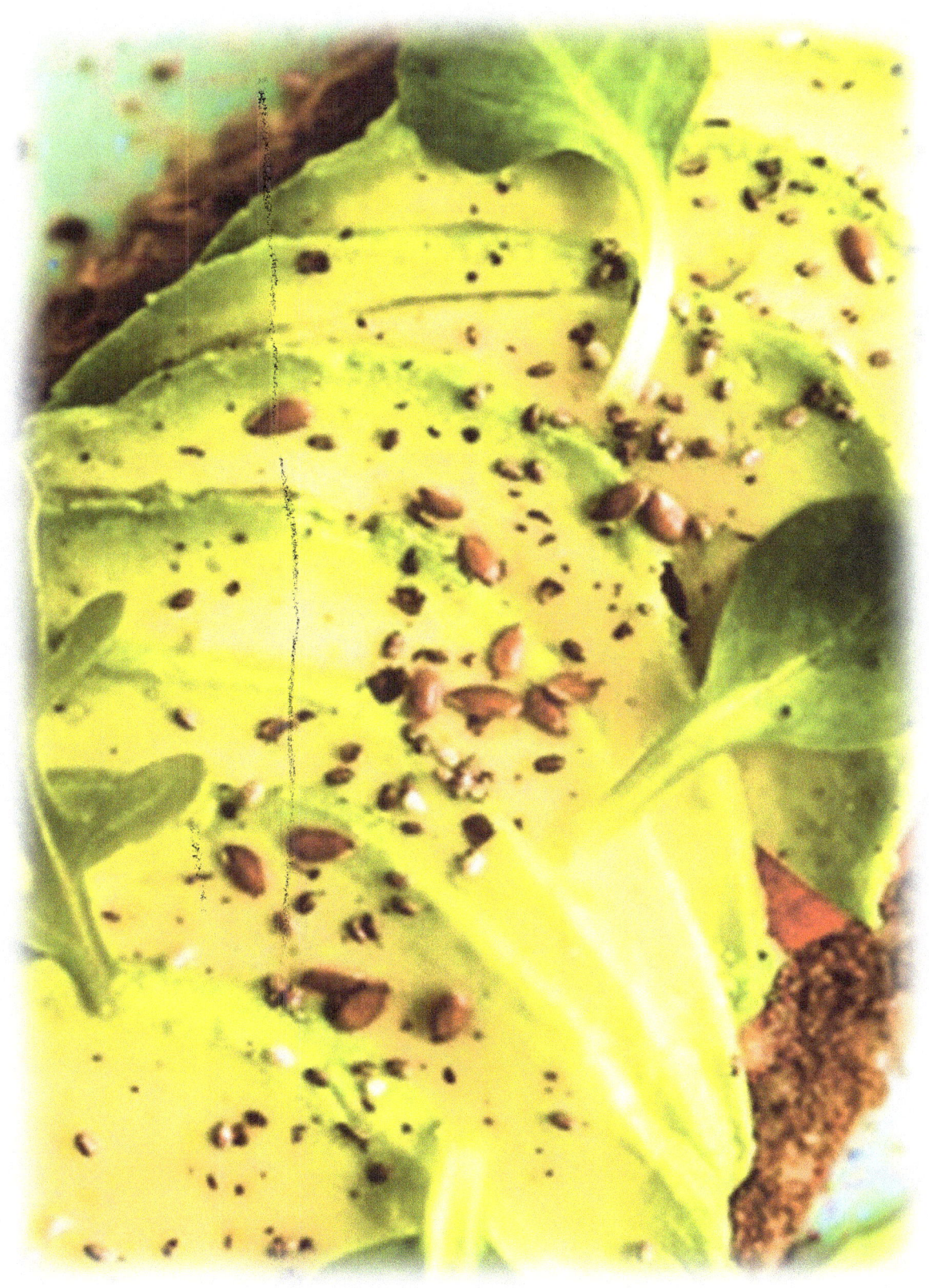

"THE RECIPES IS NO HISTORY BUT THE ART OF COOKING IS"

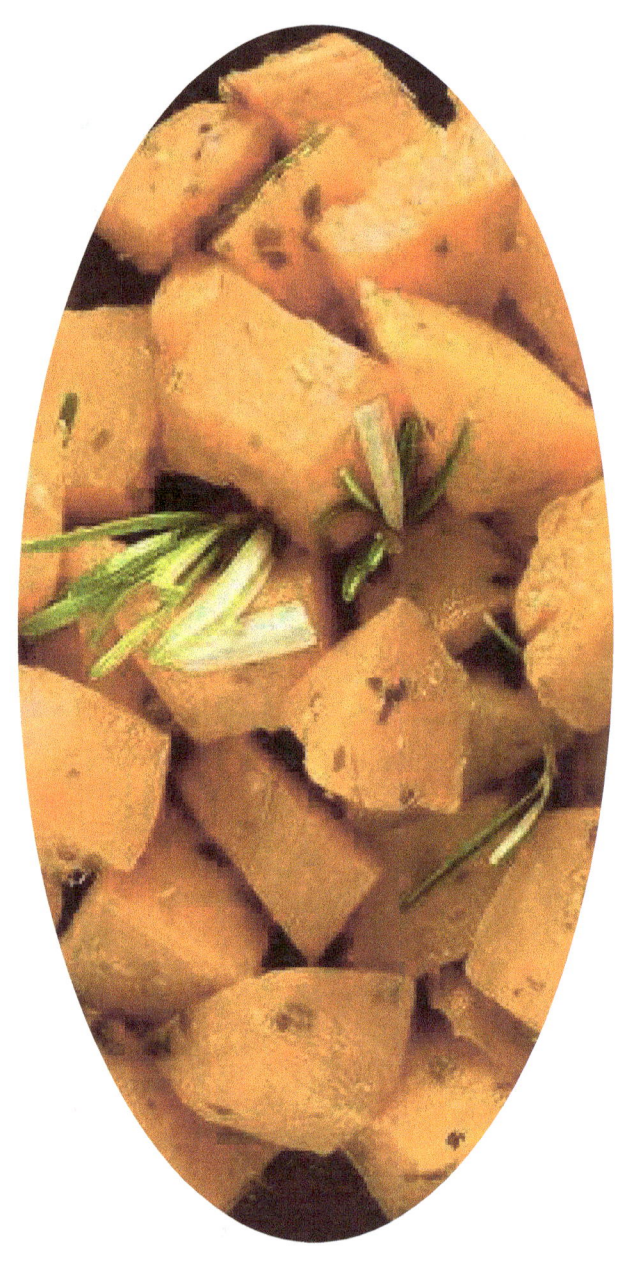

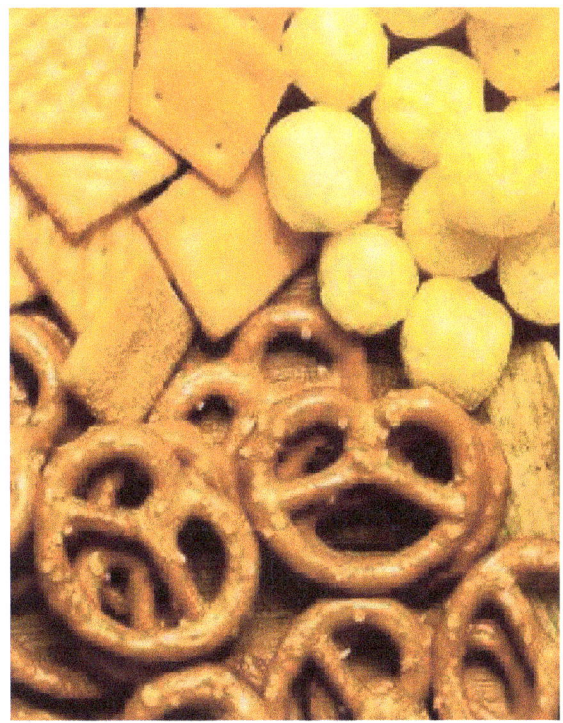

BREAKFAST RECIPES

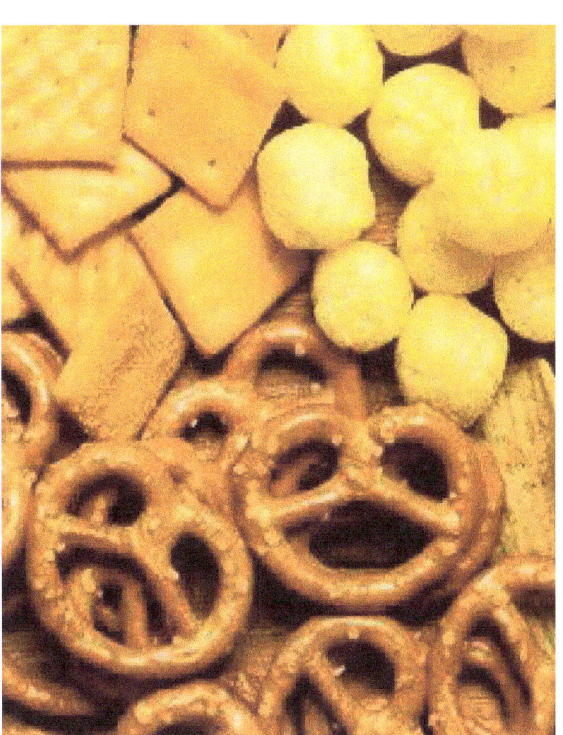

23 | LECTIN-FREE SNACKS COOKBOOK

Spicy Trail Mix

COOKING TIME: 15 minutes   **PREP TIME:** 5 minutes

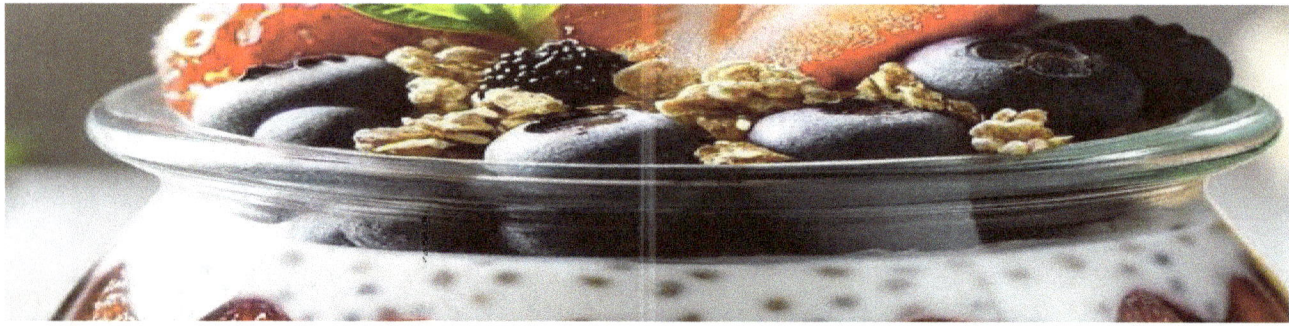

INGREDIENTS

½ cup raw almonds

¼ cup raw walnuts

¼ cup raw pumpkin seeds

2 tablespoons unsweetened dried cranberries

1 tablespoon melted coconut oil

½ teaspoon chili powder (optional)

¼ teaspoon ground cumin

Pinch of sea salt

NUTRITIONAL VALUE:
Calories: 320,
Fat: 20g,
Carbohydrates: 15g (Fiber: 3g),
Protein: 8g

PREPARATIONS

- Preheat oven to 350°F (175°C).
- In a bowl, toss almonds, walnuts, and pumpkin seeds with melted coconut oil, chili powder (optional), cumin, and sea salt.
- Spread the mixture on a baking sheet and bake for 10-12 minutes, stirring occasionally, until lightly golden brown and fragrant.
- Let cool completely.
- Combine cooled nuts and seeds with dried cranberries in a bowl.

Creamy Avocado Dip with Carrot Sticks

Portion Size: ½ cup dip with 10 baby carrots   **PREP TIME:** 5 minutes

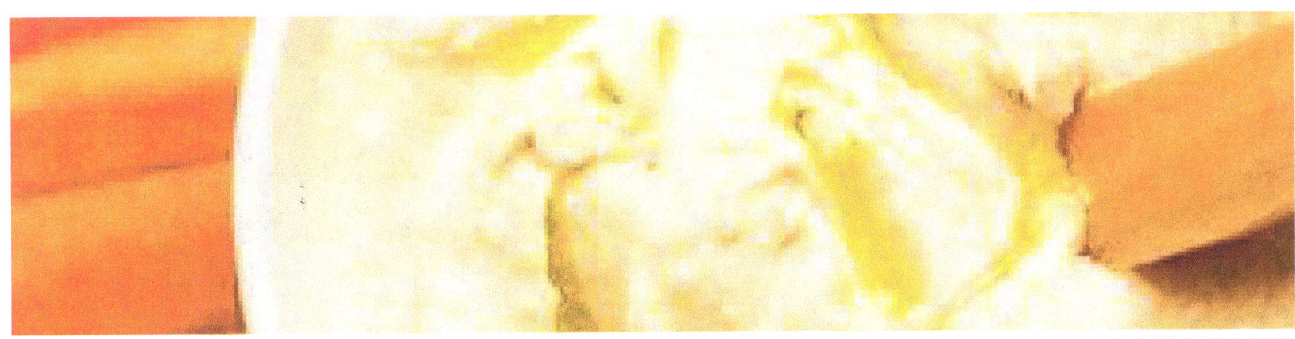

INGREDIENTS

1 ripe avocado

¼ cup chopped fresh cilantro

2 tablespoons lemon juice

1 tablespoon olive oil

¼ teaspoon sea salt

Pinch of black pepper

Baby carrots, for dipping

NUTRITIONAL VALUE:
Calories: 230,
Fat: 18g,
Carbohydrates: 7g (Fiber: 3g),
Protein: 2g

PREPARATIONS

- Halve the avocado, take out the pit, and then scoop out the flesh into a basin.
- Using a fork, mash avocado until rather chunky.
- Stir in chopped cilantro, lemon juice, olive oil, sea salt, and black pepper.
- Serve immediately with baby carrots for dipping.

Berry Bliss Smoothie

Portion Size: 1 cup   **PREP TIME:** 5 minutes

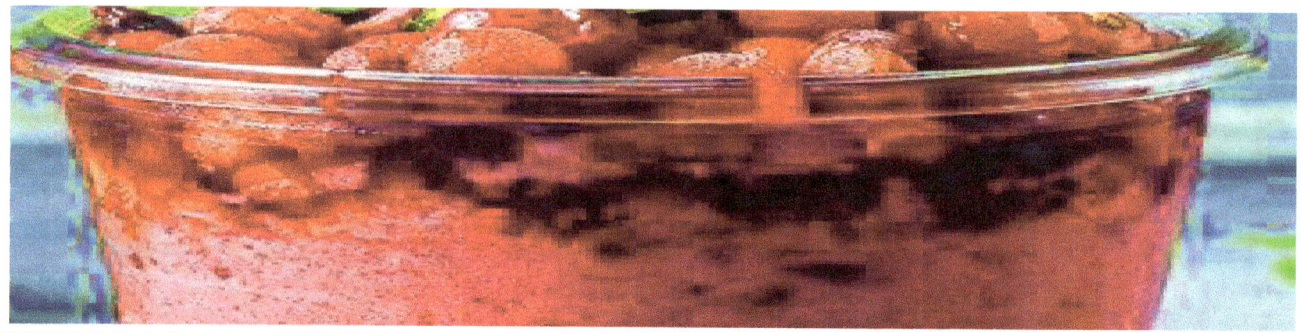

INGREDIENTS

- 1 cup frozen berries (strawberries, blueberries, raspberries)
- 1 cup unsweetened almond milk
- ½ frozen banana (optional, if tolerated)
- 1 scoop (15g) unflavored protein powder (optional)
- 1 tablespoon chia seeds
- Stevia, erythritol, or monk fruit sweetener to taste

PREPARATIONS

- Combine all ingredients in a blender.
- Blend until smooth and creamy.
- Adjust sweetness to taste with your preferred sweetener

NUTRITIONAL VALUE:

Calories: 180,

Fat: 4g,

Carbohydrates: 28g (Fiber: 7g),

Protein: 1g

Herb-Roasted Almonds

Portion Size: ¼ cup

PREP TIME: 15 minutes (including baking)

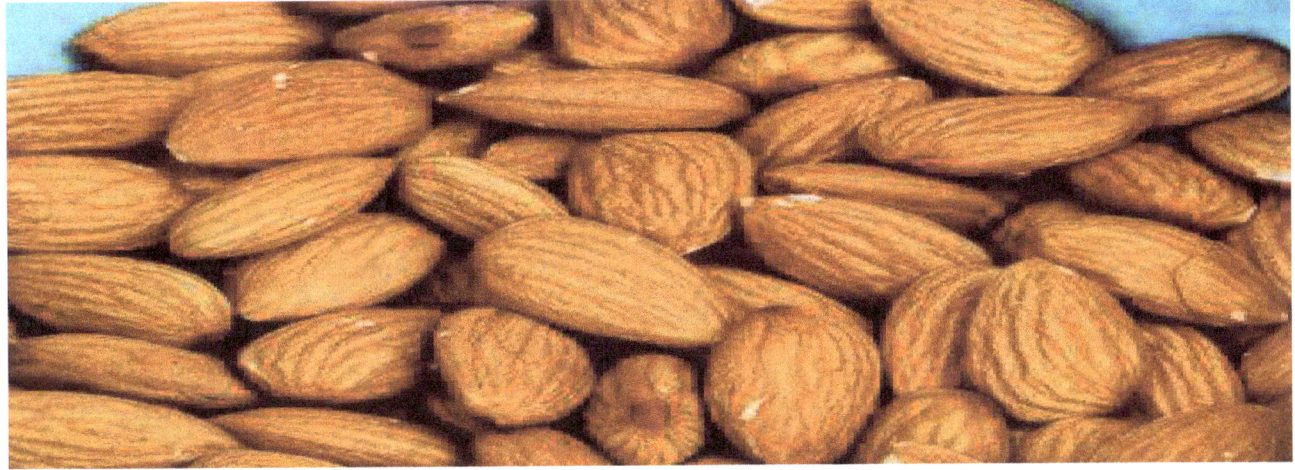

INGREDIENTS

- 1 cup raw almonds
- 1 tablespoon olive oil
- ½ teaspoon dried rosemary
- ¼ teaspoon dried thyme
- Pinch of sea salt

NUTRITIONAL VALUE:

Calories: 160,

Fat: 14g,

Carbohydrates: 6g (Fiber: 1g),

Protein: 6g

PREPARATIONS

- Preheat oven to 350°F (175°C).
- In a bowl, toss almonds with olive oil, rosemary, thyme, and sea salt.
- Spread the mixture on a baking sheet and bake for 10-12 minutes, stirring occasionally, until lightly golden brown and fragrant.
- Allow it to cool fully before putting it in an airtight container.

Zesty Cucumber Salad with Chia Seeds

Portion Size: Serves 2-3 people Total Preparation Time: 10 minutes (or 30 minutes chilled)

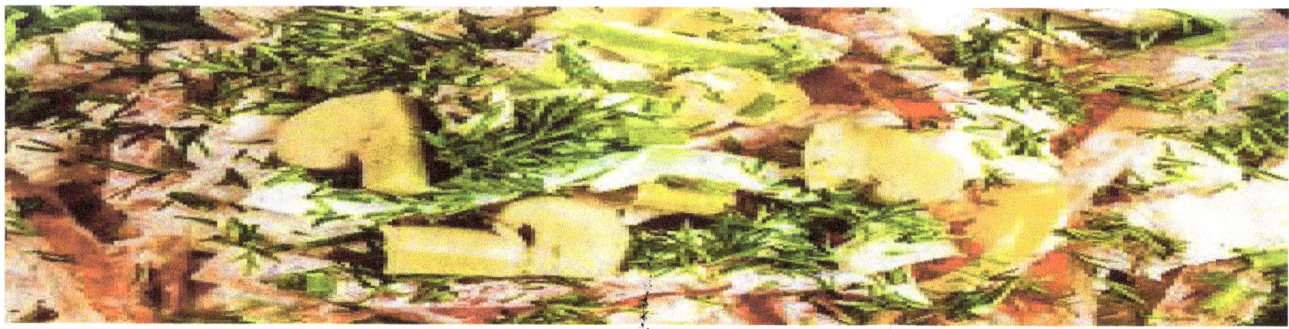

INGREDIENTS

2 large cucumbers, thinly sliced

1/4 cup chopped red onion

1/4 cup chopped fresh cilantro

1 tablespoon fresh lime juice

1 tablespoon olive oil

1 teaspoon apple cider vinegar

1/2 teaspoon Dijon mustard

1/4 teaspoon sea salt

1/4 teaspoon black pepper

2 tablespoons chia seeds

NUTRITIONAL VALUE:

Feel free to adjust the amount of red onion and cilantro to your taste preference.
For a spicier salad, add a pinch of red pepper flakes to the dressing.
You can substitute another type of vinegar, like white wine vinegar, for the apple cider vinegar.

PREPARATIONS

- In a large bowl, combine sliced cucumbers, red onion, and cilantro.
- In a small bowl, whisk together lime juice, olive oil, apple cider vinegar, Dijon mustard, salt, and pepper.
- After adding the dressing, toss the cucumber mixture to ensure even coating.
- Sprinkle chia seeds over the salad and toss gently.
- Serve immediately or refrigerate for at least 30 minutes for chilled and flavorful salad.

Nutritional Value (per serving):

Calories: 80

Fat: 4g

Carbohydrates: 7g

Fiber: 2g

Protein: 1g

Sodium: 150mg

Apple Nachos with Cinnamon-Coconut Drizzle

Portion Size: Serves 2-3 people   **PREP TIME:** 10 minutes

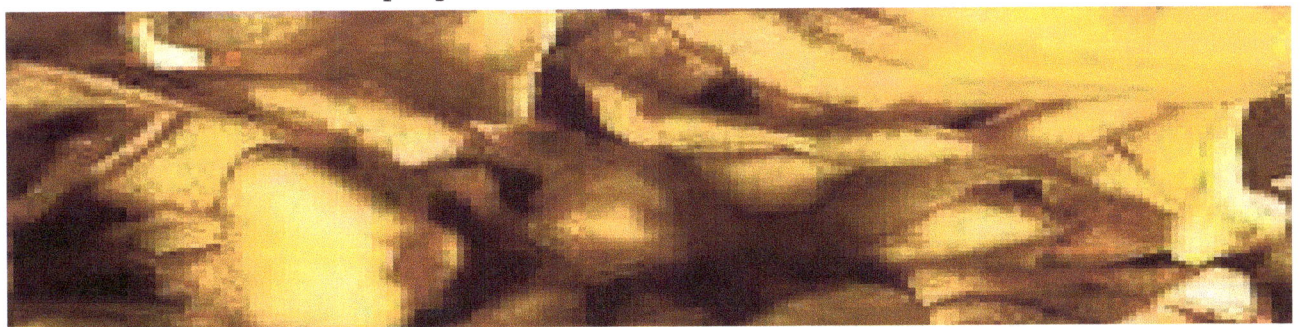

INGREDIENTS

1/4 cup unsweetened shredded coconut
1/4 cup chopped walnuts
1/4 cup chopped pecans
1/4 cup chopped dried cranberries (unsweetened)
2 tablespoons melted coconut oil
1 tablespoon ground cinnamon
1 tablespoon honey

Notes:

You can use any type of nut or dried fruit that you prefer.

For a vegan option, omit the honey and use agave nectar or maple syrup as a substitute.

If the coconut oil solidifies, simply reheat it slightly to liquefy it again.

PREPARATIONS

- Arrange apple slices on a plate or serving platter in a single layer.
- In a small saucepan, combine melted coconut oil, cinnamon, and honey. Heat over low heat, stirring constantly, until well combined and fragrant.
- Sprinkle the chopped nuts, coconut, and dried cranberries over the apple slices.
- Drizzle the warm cinnamon-coconut drizzle over the top of the apple nachos.

NUTRITIONAL VALUE:

Calories: 350
Fat: 18g
Carbohydrates: 40g
Fiber: 6g
Protein: 4g
Sodium: 30mg

Mini Frittata Cups with Broccoli and Cheddar

Portion Size: Makes 6 mini frittatas **PREP TIME:** 15 minutes

INGREDIENTS

- 6 eggs
- 1/2 cup chopped broccoli florets (steamed)
- 1/4 cup shredded cheddar cheese (optional)
- 1/4 cup chopped red onion
- 1/4 cup chopped fresh mushrooms
- 1 tablespoon chopped fresh parsley
- 1/4 teaspoon dried oregano
- Salt and black pepper to taste
- Cooking spray or olive oil

Notes:

You can add other vegetables like chopped spinach, bell peppers, or zucchini to these frittatas.

If you don't have fresh herbs, you can use 1/2 teaspoon dried parsley instead. For a vegetarian option, omit the cheddar cheese.

These mini frittatas can be stored in an airtight container in the refrigerator for up to 3 days. Reheat in the microwave for a quick and easy breakfast or snack.

PREPARATIONS

- Preheat oven to 375°F (190°C). Apply cooking spray or olive oil to a muffin pan to make it greasy.
- In a large bowl, whisk together eggs, parsley, oregano, salt, and pepper.
- Fold in the steamed broccoli florets, chopped red onion, mushrooms, and shredded cheddar cheese (if using).
- Spoon the egg mixture evenly into each muffin cup that has been oiled.
- Fry for 15 to 20 minutes, or until the frittatas are cooked through and have a golden brown crust.
- Let cool slightly before serving.

NUTRITIONAL VALUE:

Calories: 100
- Fat: 7g
- Carbohydrates: 2g
- Fiber: 1g
- Protein: 7g
- Sodium: 80mg

No-Bake Energy Bites with Dates and Walnuts

COOKING TIME: minutes **PREP TIME:** minutes

INGREDIENTS

- 1 cup pitted medjool dates
- 1/2 cup chopped walnuts
- 1/4 cup unsweetened shredded coconut (plus extra for coating)
- 2 tablespoons rolled oats
- 1 tablespoon chia seeds
- 1 teaspoon ground cinnamon
- Pinch of sea salt

NUTRITIONAL VALUE:

Calories: 180
Fat: 8g
Carbohydrates: 25g
Fiber: 3g
Protein: 2g
Sodium: 30mg

PREPARATIONS

- In a food processor, pulse the pitted dates until they become a sticky paste.
- Add the chopped walnuts, shredded coconut (reserving some for coating), rolled oats, chia seeds, cinnamon, and salt.
- Pulse the mixture until it combines well and forms a cohesive dough.
- With your hands, roll the dough into bite-sized balls.
- Coat each ball with the remaining shredded coconut.
- Place the energy bites on a plate or baking sheet lined with parchment paper.
- Refrigerate for at least 30 minutes to allow them to harden.

Tropical Fruit Skewers with Lime and Mint

Portion Size: Makes 2-3 skewers   **PREP TIME:** 10 minutes

INGREDIENTS

- 1 cup assorted fresh tropical fruits (such as pineapple chunks, mango chunks, kiwi slices, papaya chunks)
- 1/2 lime, juiced
- 1 tablespoon honey
- 1 tablespoon chopped fresh mint leaves
- Wooden skewers

NUTRITIONAL VALUE:

Calories: 80
Fat: 0g
Carbohydrates: 20g
Fiber: 2g
Protein: 0g
Sodium: 2mg

PREPARATIONS

- Wash and cut the fresh tropical fruits into bite-sized pieces.
- In a small bowl, whisk together lime juice and honey.
- Add the chopped mint leaves to the lime-honey mixture.
- Thread the fruit pieces onto wooden skewers, alternating different types of fruits for a visually appealing presentation.
- Brush the fruit skewers lightly with the lime-honey-mint mixture.

Notes:
You can use any type of fresh fruit that you like on these skewers. Other good options include strawberries, blueberries, and grapes.
If you don't have fresh mint, you can use a sprinkle of dried mint instead.

Simple Green Salad with Lemon Vinaigrette

Portion Size: Serves 2 people **PREP TIME:** 10 minutes

INGREDIENTS

- 4 cups mixed greens (such as romaine, spinach, or baby kale)
- 1/2 cup cherry tomatoes, halved
- 1/4 cup sliced cucumber
- 1/4 cup crumbled feta cheese (optional)
- 2 tablespoons olive oil
- 1 tablespoon fresh lemon juice
- 1 teaspoon Dijon mustard
- 1/2 teaspoon honey
- Salt and black pepper to taste

NUTRITIONAL VALUE:

- Calories: 150
- Fat: 10g
- Carbohydrates: 10g
- Fiber: 2g
- Protein: 2g
- Sodium: 60mg

PREPARATIONS

- In a large bowl, combine the mixed greens, cherry tomatoes, and sliced cucumber.
- In a small jar or bowl, whisk together olive oil, lemon juice, Dijon mustard, honey, salt, and pepper.
- Drizzle the salad with the vinaigrette and toss to coat evenly.
- Top with crumbled feta cheese (if using) and serve immediately.

"FOOD AND COOKING REMAINS THE MOST NATURAL HEALER"

Nutrient-Packed Lectin-Free Snacks for Energy

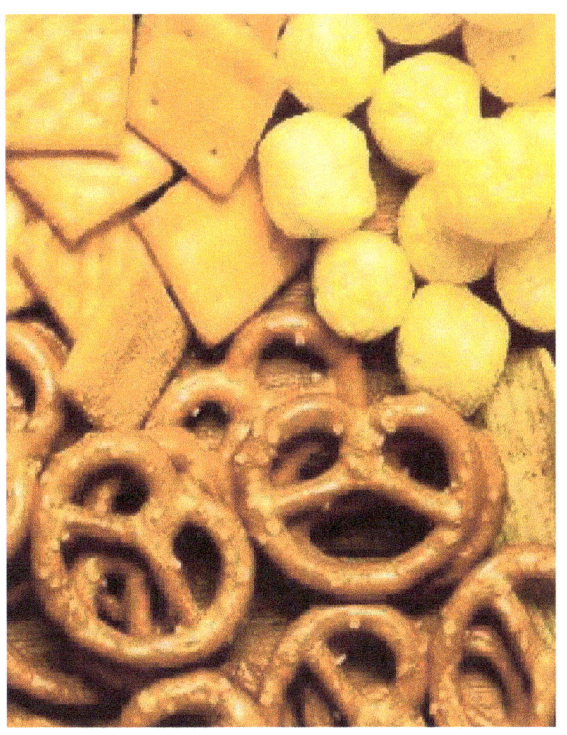
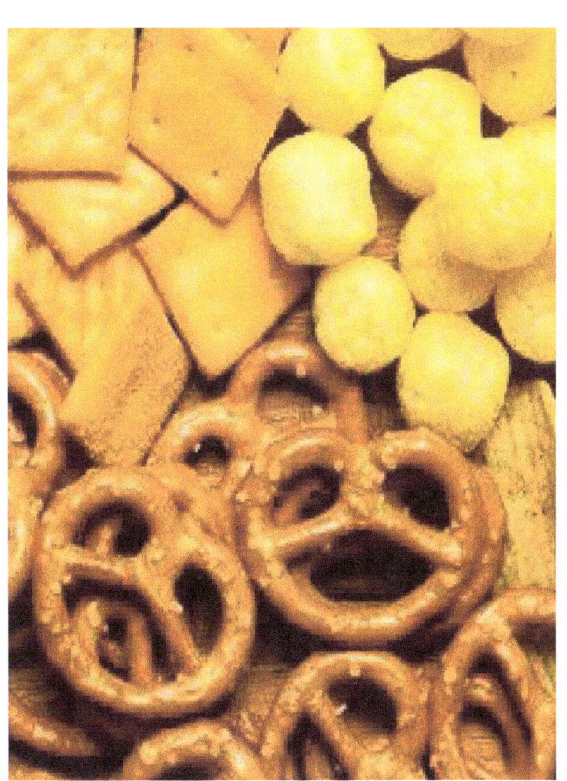

35 | LECTIN-FREE SNACKS COOKBOOK

Power Veggie Sticks with Creamy Avocado Dip

Portion Size: Serves 2-3 people

PREP TIME: 10 minutes

INGREDIENTS

For the Veggie Sticks:

- 2 large carrots, peeled and cut into sticks
- 1 large cucumber, peeled and cut into sticks
- 1 bell pepper (optional, if tolerated), sliced
- 1 cup celery stalks, cut into sticks
- 1 zucchini, sliced (optional)

For the Creamy Avocado Dip:

- 1 ripe avocado
- 1/4 cup chopped fresh cilantro
- 1 tablespoon fresh lime juice
- 1 tablespoon olive oil
- 1/4 teaspoon sea salt
- 1/4 teaspoon black pepper

PREPARATIONS

- Prepare the Veggie Sticks: Wash and chop the vegetables into sticks or desired shapes. Arrange them on a serving platter.
- Make the Creamy Avocado Dip:
- In a food processor or blender, combine the avocado flesh, chopped cilantro, lime juice, olive oil, salt, and pepper. Blend until smooth and creamy.
- Serve:
- Transfer the avocado dip to a small bowl and place it next to the veggie sticks on the serving platter. Enjoy!

NUTRITIONAL VALUE:

Calories: 150
Fat: 10g
Carbohydrates: 10g
Fiber: 5g
Protein: 2g
Sodium: 120mg

Notes:
Feel free to adjust the amount of lime juice and spices to your taste preference.
You can substitute another herb, such as parsley, for the cilantro.
For a thicker dip, add a tablespoon of chopped cooked chickpeas (optional, if tolerated).

Berry Bliss Smoothie Bowl

Portion Size: 1 serving   **PREP TIME:** 5 minutes

INGREDIENTS

- 1 cup frozen berries (mixed berries, blueberries, strawberries, etc.)
- 1/2 cup unsweetened almond milk (or other plant-based milk)
- 1/2 banana, frozen (optional)
- 1 tablespoon unsweetened shredded coconut
- 1 scoop green powder (optional)
- 1/2 teaspoon stevia or monk fruit sweetener (optional)

NUTRITIONAL VALUE:

- Calories: 200
- Fat: 5g
- Carbohydrates: 30g
- Fiber: 5g
- Protein: 2g
- Sodium: 30mg

PREPARATIONS

- In a blender, combine frozen berries, almond milk, frozen banana (if using), shredded coconut, green powder (if using), and sweetener (if using).
- Blend until smooth and creamy.
- Pour the smoothie into a bowl.

Notes:

You can use any type of frozen berries that you prefer.

If you don't have frozen banana, you can use a few ice cubes instead.

To suit your taste, change the amount of sweetener.

Feel free to add other toppings to your smoothie bowl, such as granola, chopped nuts, or chia seeds.

Spiced Nut & Seed Trail Mix

Portion Size: 1 serving   **PREP TIME:** 5 minutes

INGREDIENTS

- 1/2 cup raw almonds
- 1/4 cup raw walnuts
- 1/4 cup raw pumpkin seeds (pepitas)
- 2 tablespoons hemp seeds (optional)
- 1/4 cup unsweetened dried cranberries
- 1/4 teaspoon ground cinnamon
- 1/8 teaspoon ground ginger (optional)

PREPARATIONS

- In a large bowl, combine almonds, walnuts, pumpkin seeds, hemp seeds (if using), dried cranberries, cinnamon, and ginger (if using).
- Toss to coat evenly.

NUTRITIONAL VALUE:

- Calories: 300
- Fat: 15g
- Carbohydrates: 20g
- Fiber: 5g
- Protein: 8g
- Sodium: 30mg

Notes:
- You can use any type of nuts and seeds that you prefer.
- For a sweeter trail mix, you can add a few chopped dates or dried figs.
- Store the trail mix in an airtight container at room temperature for up to a week.

Crispy Coconut Chips with Citrus Dip

Portion Size: Makes about 2 cups of chips (serves 4-6)

PREP TIME: 10 minutes

INGREDIENTS

For the Chips:

2 cups unsweetened shredded coconut flakes

1 tablespoon melted coconut oil

1/4 teaspoon sea salt

For the Dip (choose one option):

Option 1: Yogurt Dip:

1/2 cup plain Greek yogurt (optional, if tolerated)

1 tablespoon fresh lime juice

1/4 teaspoon honey (or maple syrup for vegan option)

Pinch of ground ginger

NUTRITIONAL VALUE:

Calories: 180
Fat: 14g
Carbohydrates: 12g
Fiber: 2g
Protein: 2g
Sodium: 40mg

PREPARATIONS

- Preheat oven to 350°F (175°C). Line a baking sheet with parchment paper.
- In a large bowl, toss the coconut flakes with melted coconut oil and sea salt until evenly coated.
- Spread the coconut flakes in a single layer on the prepared baking sheet.
- Bake for 10-15 minutes, stirring occasionally, until golden brown and crispy. Be careful not to burn them.
- While the chips are baking, prepare your chosen dip option (see below).
- For Yogurt Dip: Whisk together Greek yogurt, lime juice, honey (or maple syrup), and ground ginger in a small bowl.
- For Mango Dip: Blend together chopped mango, coconut milk, lime juice, and ground cinnamon in a blender or food processor until smooth.
- Let the coconut chips cool slightly before serving with the chosen dip.

Zucchini Noodle Primavera

Portion Size: Serves 2 **PREP TIME:** 15 minutes

INGREDIENTS

- 2 medium zucchinis
- 1 tablespoon olive oil
- 1 clove garlic, minced
- 1/2 cup chopped red onion
- 1 cup chopped broccoli florets (steamed)
- 1/2 cup sliced mushrooms
- 1/4 cup chopped cherry tomatoes
- 1/4 cup chopped fresh parsley
- 1/4 teaspoon dried oregano
- Salt and black pepper to taste
- 1/4 cup grated Parmesan cheese

NUTRITIONAL VALUE:

- Calories: 200
- Fat: 8g
- Carbohydrates: 20g
- Fiber: 4g
- Protein: 5g
- Sodium: 150mg

PREPARATIONS

- Using a spiralizer or julienne peeler, spiralize the zucchinis into noodles.
- In a big skillet over medium heat, warm up the olive oil. Add garlic and red onion, and cook until softened, about 3 minutes.
- Add the broccoli, mushrooms, and cherry tomatoes to the pan and cook for another 5 minutes, or until the vegetables are tender-crisp.
- Add the zucchini noodles to the pan and toss to combine. Cook for an additional 2-3 minutes, or until the noodles are heated through.
- Stir in the chopped parsley and oregano. Season with salt and pepper to taste.
- Serve immediately, topped with grated Parmesan cheese (optional).

Apple Slices with Almond Butter

Portion Size: Serves 1-2 people   **PREP TIME: 15** minutes

INGREDIENTS

- 2 large apples (such as Gala, Honeycrisp, or Fuji)
- 1/4 cup natural almond butter (creamy or crunchy)
- Optional: Ground cinnamon for sprinkling

NUTRITIONAL VALUE:

- Calories: 320
- Fat: 18g
- Carbohydrates: 38g
- Fiber: 8g
- Protein: 6g
- Sodium: 30mg

PREPARATIONS

- Wash and dry the apples. Cut them into bite-sized pieces or thin slices, depending on your choice.
- Spoon the almond butter into a small bowl for easy dipping.
- Preparation Time: 5 minutes

Notes:
- For a sweeter option, choose a sweeter apple variety like Fuji.
- If the almond butter is too thick for dipping, add a teaspoon of honey or maple syrup (optional) to thin it slightly.
- Sprinkle ground cinnamon over the apple slices for an extra flavor boost.
- Other nut butters like cashew butter or sunflower seed butter (optional, if tolerated) can be used as a substitute for almond butter.

Frittata Bites with Fresh Herbs

Portion Size: Makes 6-8 frittata bites   **PREP TIME:** 10 minutes

INGREDIENTS

- 4 eggs
- 1/4 cup chopped vegetables (such as broccoli, bell peppers, mushrooms, or spinach)
- 1/4 cup shredded cheese (optional)
- 1 tablespoon chopped fresh herbs (such as parsley, basil, or chives)
- Salt and black pepper to taste
- Cooking spray or olive oil

NUTRITIONAL VALUE:

Calories: 50
Fat: 4g
Carbohydrates: 1g
Fiber: 0.5g
Protein: 4g
Sodium: 60mg

PREPARATIONS

- Preheat oven to 375°F (190°C). Lightly grease a mini muffin tin with cooking spray or olive oil.
- In a medium bowl, whisk together eggs, chopped vegetables, shredded cheese (if using), and fresh herbs. To taste, add salt and pepper for seasoning.
- Evenly divide the egg mixture among the muffin cups that have been oiled.
- Bake the frittatas for 15 to 20 minutes, or until they are set and have a golden brown top.
- Let cool slightly before serving.

Pear and Pecan Energy Balls

Portion Size: Makes approximately 10-12 energy balls

PREP TIME: 15 minutes

INGREDIENTS

- 1 cup pitted medjool dates
- 1 cup chopped pecans
- 1/2 cup chopped pear
- 1/4 cup unsweetened shredded coconut
- 2 tablespoons ground cinnamon
- 1 tablespoon chia seeds

NUTRITIONAL VALUE:

- **Calories:** 220
- **Fat:** 12g
- **Carbohydrates:** 30g
- **Fiber:** 4g
- **Protein:** 3g
- **Sodium:** 20mg

PREPARATIONS

- In a food processor, pulse the medjool dates until they become a sticky paste.
- Add the chopped pecans, pear, shredded coconut, cinnamon, and chia seeds to the food processor. Pulse the ingredients until a dough develops and they are well blended.
- Using your hands, roll the mixture into bite-sized balls.
- For up to a week, keep the energy balls refrigerated in an airtight container.

Notes:

Add a spoonful of water or almond milk to the mixture if it's too dry to work together.

You can substitute other dried fruits like raisins or cranberries (unsweetened) for the pear.

To prevent sticking, you can roll the energy balls in additional shredded coconut or chopped nuts.

Pumpkin Seed & Celery Seed Hummus

Portion Size: Makes about 1 1/2 cups of hummus   **PREP TIME:** 10 minutes

INGREDIENTS

- One can (15 oz) of rinsed and drained chickpeas
- 1/2 cup raw pumpkin seeds
- 2 tablespoons tahini (sesame seed paste)
- 2 tablespoons olive oil
- 1/4 cup lemon juice
- 1/4 cup water
- 1 teaspoon ground cumin
- 1/2 teaspoon dried oregano
- 1/2 teaspoon garlic powder
- 1/4 teaspoon sea salt
- 1/4 teaspoon black pepper
- 1 teaspoon celery seeds

PREPARATIONS

- In a food processor, combine the drained and rinsed chickpeas, raw pumpkin seeds, tahini, olive oil, lemon juice, water, cumin, oregano, garlic powder, salt, and pepper.
- Scoop down the sides as necessary and process until creamy and smooth.
- Add the celery seeds and pulse a few more times to incorporate them.
- Taste and adjust seasonings as desired.
- Serve the hummus with sliced vegetables, cucumber sticks, or pita bread for dipping.

NUTRITIONAL VALUE:
Calories: 120
Fat: 7g
Carbohydrates: 10g
Fiber: 2g
Protein: 4g
Sodium: 180mg

Spiced Melon Skewers with Coconut Yogurt Dip

Portion Size: Makes about 4-6 skewers and 1 cup of dip

PREP TIME: 15 minutes

INGREDIENTS

For the Skewers:
1 cantaloupe, cut into bite-sized cubes
1 honeydew melon, cut into bite-sized cubes
1/4 cup fresh mint leaves, chopped (optional)

For the Dip:
1 cup plain coconut yogurt (unsweetened)
1/4 cup chopped fresh mango (optional)
1 tablespoon honey
1/2 teaspoon ground ginger
1/4 teaspoon ground cinnamon
Pinch of ground cardamom (optional)

NUTRITIONAL VALUE:

Calories: 150

Fat: 3g

Carbohydrates: 25g

Fiber: 2g

Protein: 2g

Sodium: 20mg

NOTE

You can substitute other types of melon for the cantaloupe and honeydew, such as watermelon or galia melon.

If you don't have fresh mango, you can use another type of fruit like pineapple or papaya.

PREPARATIONS

For the Skewers:

Thread the cantaloupe and honeydew melon cubes onto skewers, alternating colors for a visually appealing presentation.

If using, gently fold in the chopped fresh mint leaves between the melon cubes.

For the Dip:

In a small bowl, whisk together the coconut yogurt, chopped mango (if using), honey, ginger, cinnamon, and cardamom (if using).

If the dip is too thick, add a tablespoon or two of milk or water to thin it out to your desired consistency.

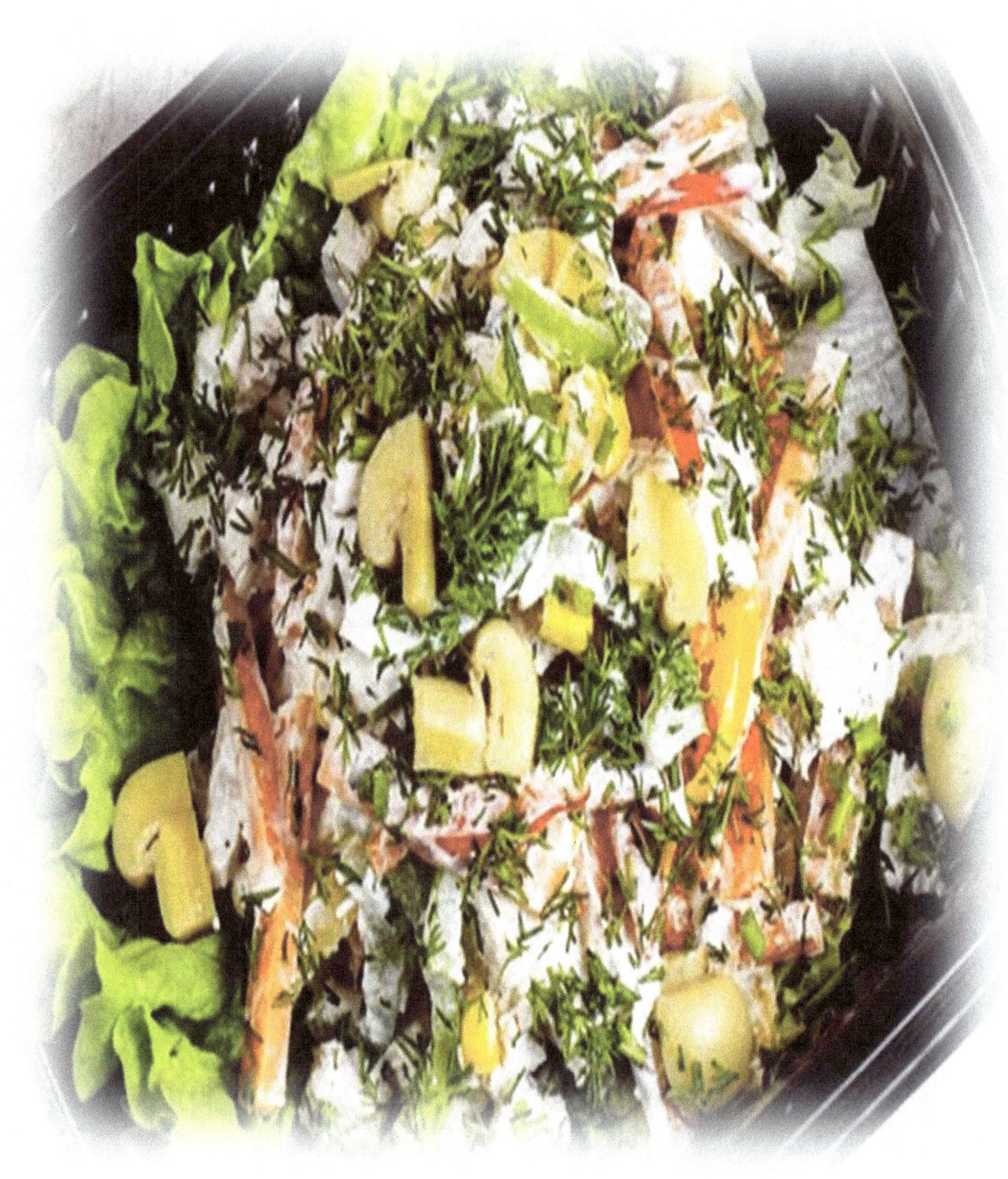

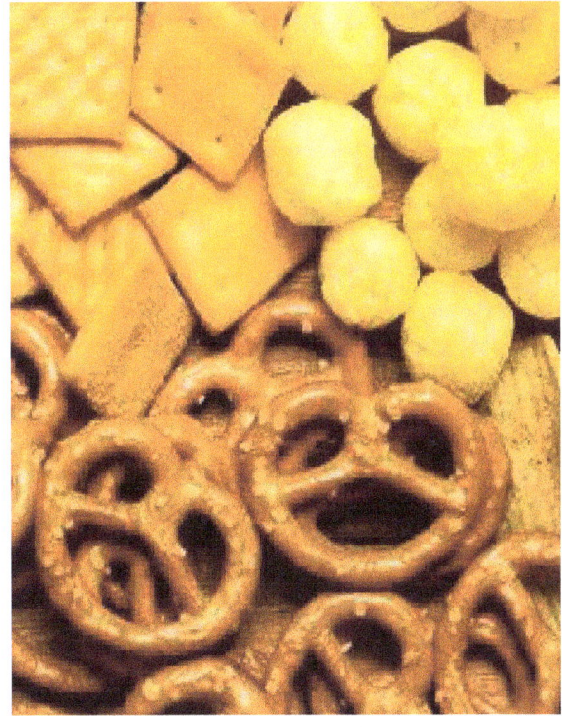

Creative Lectin-Free Snacks for Every Occasion

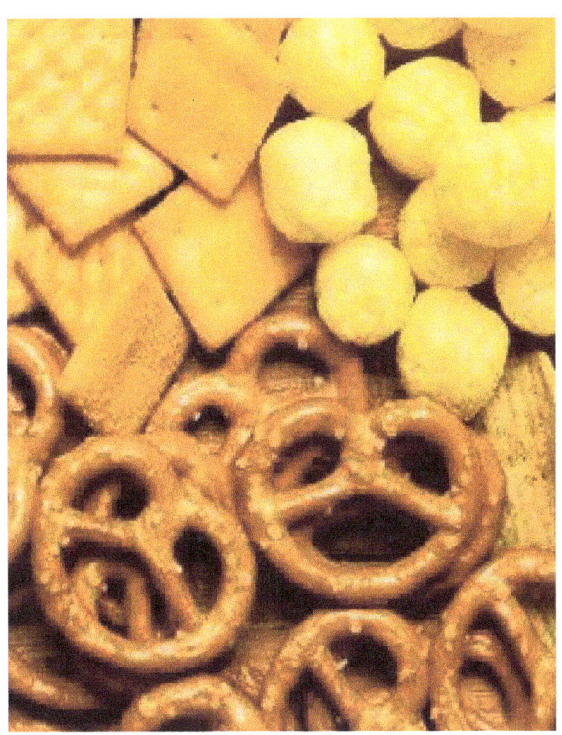

47 | LECTIN-FREE SNACKS COOKBOOK

Elegant Caprese Skewers with Balsamic Glaze

Portion Size: Serves 4-6 people **PREP TIME: 10 minutes**

INGREDIENTS

- 1 pint cherry tomatoes (smaller are preferable)
- Eight ounces of fresh mozzarella balls, the size of pearls or ciliegine
- 1 bunch fresh basil, leaves removed from stem
- 2-4 tablespoons balsamic glaze (store-bought or homemade)

NUTRITIONAL VALUE:

- Calories: 80
- Fat: 4g
- Carbohydrates: 7g
- Fiber: 1g
- Protein: 4g
- Sodium: 180mg

PREPARATIONS

- Wash and dry cherry tomatoes. If using larger tomatoes, halve them.
- Thread a mozzarella ball, a basil leaf (folded in half or thirds if large), and a cherry tomato onto a toothpick or small skewer. Repeat to create as many skewers as desired.
- Arrange the skewers on a serving platter.
- When ready to serve, drizzle the skewers with the balsamic glaze.

Notes:

For a more flavorful option, marinate the cherry tomatoes in a drizzle of olive oil, balsamic vinegar, and a pinch of salt and pepper for 30 minutes before assembling the skewers.

You can use a variety of fresh herbs like parsley or oregano instead of basil.

If you don't have balsamic glaze, you can reduce balsamic vinegar in a saucepan over low heat until thickened.

Mini Bell Pepper Poppers Stuffed with Cashew Cheese

Portion Size: Serves 6-8 people (2 halves per person)

PREP TIME: 45 minutes

INGREDIENTS

Three huge bell peppers (yellow, orange, or red)

One cup of uncooked cashews, soaking for two hours or overnight

1/2 cup nutritional yeast

1/4 cup chopped red onion

2 tablespoons lemon juice

1 tablespoon olive oil

1 teaspoon dried oregano

1/2 teaspoon garlic powder

1/4 teaspoon smoked paprika (optional)

Salt and black pepper to taste

NUTRITIONAL VALUE:

Calories: 150, Fat: 9g
Carbohydrates: 15g, Fiber: 2g
Protein: 5g, Sodium: 30mg

PREPARATIONS

- Preheat oven to 375°F (190°C). Line a baking sheet with parchment paper.
- Remove the seeds and membranes from the bell peppers by cutting them in half lengthwise.
- In a high-powered blender or food processor, combine soaked cashews, nutritional yeast, red onion, lemon juice, olive oil, oregano, garlic powder, smoked paprika (if using), salt, and pepper. Blend until smooth and creamy.
- Stuff the bell pepper halves with the cashew cheese mixture.
- Bake for 20-25 minutes, or until the bell peppers are tender and the filling is slightly golden brown.
- Let cool slightly before serving.

Festive Guacamole Cups with Plantain Chips

Portion Size: Serves 4 people　　**PREP TIME: 10** minutes

INGREDIENTS

- 2 ripe avocados, halved, pitted, and flesh scooped out
- 1/4 cup chopped red onion
- 1/4 cup chopped fresh cilantro
- 1 tablespoon fresh lime juice
- 1/2 teaspoon ground cumin
- 1/4 teaspoon chili powder (optional)
- 1/4 teaspoon sea salt
- 1/4 teaspoon black pepper
- 1/4 cup cherry tomatoes, halved (optional)
- 1/4 cup crumbled cotija cheese (optional)
- 1 bag (around 6 oz) baked plantain chips

PREPARATIONS

- In a medium bowl, mash the avocado flesh with a fork until slightly chunky.
- Stir in the chopped red onion, cilantro, lime juice, cumin, chili powder (optional), salt, and pepper.
- Gently fold in the halved cherry tomatoes (optional) and crumbled cotija cheese (optional).
- Divide the guacamole mixture evenly amongst 4 small serving cups or ramekins.
- Serve immediately with baked plantain chips for scooping.

NUTRITIONAL VALUE:

Calories: 250

Fat: 18g

Carbohydrates: 15g

Fiber: 7g

Protein: 2g

Sodium: 180mg

Savory Mushroom and Spinach Pinwheels for Party Platters

Portion Size: Makes about 20-24 pinwheels   **PREP TIME:** 20 minutes

INGREDIENTS

- One sheet of frozen puff pastry, thawed according package directions
- 1 tablespoon olive oil
- 1 small onion, diced
- 8 oz sliced mushrooms (cremini, portobello, or a mix)
- 4 cups fresh spinach, roughly chopped
- 1/4 cup crumbled feta cheese
- 1/4 cup shredded mozzarella cheese
- 1/4 teaspoon dried oregano
- 1/4 teaspoon garlic powder
- Salt and black pepper to taste
- 1 egg, beaten with 1 tablespoon water (egg wash)

PREPARATION

- Preheat oven to 400°F (200°C). Line a baking sheet with parchment paper.
- In a big skillet over medium heat, warm up the olive oil. Cook for approximately five minutes, or until the diced onion is tender.
- Add the sliced mushrooms to the skillet and cook until browned and softened, about 7 minutes.
- Add the chopped spinach and simmer for about two minutes, or until it wilts.

PREPARATIONS

Drain any excess liquid from the spinach mixture.

- In a medium bowl, combine the cooked mushroom and spinach mixture, crumbled feta cheese, shredded mozzarella cheese, oregano, garlic powder, salt, and pepper.
- Spread a thin layer of flour on a surface and unfold the sheet of thawed puff pastry. Roll out the puff pastry slightly to form a rectangle.
- Spread the prepared mushroom and spinach filling evenly over the entire surface of the puff pastry sheet, leaving a 1-inch border at the long edge.
- Starting from the long edge with the filling, roll up the puff pastry dough tightly into a log shape. Pinch the seam to seal.
- Brush the top of the pastry roll with the egg wash.
- Using a sharp knife, carefully cut the pastry roll into 1-inch slices. As soon as the baking sheet is ready, place the pinwheels cut side down.
- Puff and get golden brown after 20 to 25 minutes of baking.
- Let cool slightly before serving.

"A DESERT A DAY PERFECTS THE DAY"

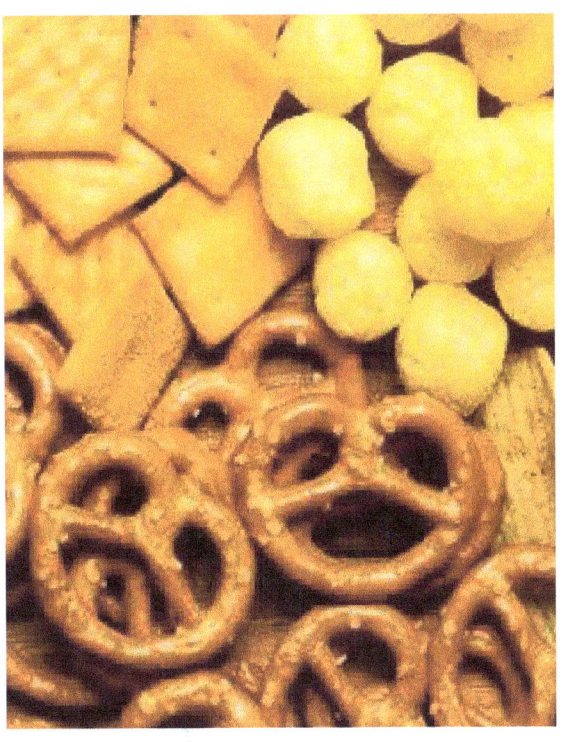

Decadent Desserts Sans Lectins

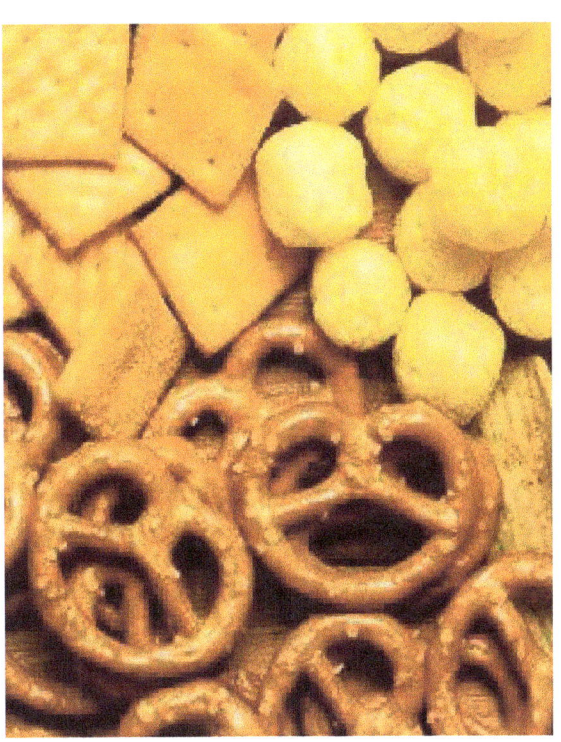

Spiced Berry Crumble with Coconut Topping

Portion Size: Serves 4-6 people

PREP TIME: 15 minutes

INGREDIENTS

For the Fruit Filling:
2 cups mixed berries (strawberries, blueberries, raspberries)
1 tablespoon arrowroot flour (optional)
1/4 cup water
1/4 cup chopped pecans
1 tablespoon lemon juice
1/4 teaspoon ground cinnamon
Pinch of sea salt

For the Coconut Topping:
1/2 cup almond flour
1/4 cup shredded coconut (unsweetened)
1/4 cup chopped pecans
2 tablespoons melted coconut oil
1/4 teaspoon ground cinnamon
Pinch of sea salt

NUTRITIONAL VALUE:

Calories: 300 (approximate)
Fat: 15g (approximate)
Carbohydrates: 25g (approximate)
Fiber: 4g (approximate)
Protein: 4g (approximate)
Sodium: 50mg (approximate)

PREPARATIONS

- Preheat oven to 375°F (190°C). Lightly grease a small baking dish (around 8x8 inches).
- Prepare the Fruit Filling: In a bowl, combine the mixed berries, arrowroot flour (optional), water, chopped pecans, lemon juice, cinnamon, and sea salt. Toss to coat the berries evenly.
- into the baking dish that has been ready, pour the berry mixture..
- Make the Coconut Topping: In a separate bowl, combine the almond flour, shredded coconut, chopped pecans, melted coconut oil, cinnamon, and sea salt. Crumble together using a fork or your fingertips..
- Sprinkle the coconut topping evenly over the berry mixture in the baking dish.
- Bake for 25-30 minutes, or until the fruit filling is bubbly and the topping is golden brown.
- Let cool slightly before serving.

Creamy Avocado Mousse with Citrus Glaze

Portion Size: Serves 2 people   **PREP TIME:** 10 minutes

INGREDIENTS

- For the Avocado Mousse:
- Two ripe avocados with the flesh removed and pitted
- 1/4 cup unsweetened almond milk
- 2 tablespoons fresh lime juice
- 1 tablespoon honey or maple syrup
- 1/2 teaspoon vanilla extract
- Pinch of sea salt
- For the Citrus Glaze (Optional):
- 2 tablespoons orange juice
- 1 tablespoon lemon juice
- 1 tablespoon honey or maple syrup

NUTRITIONAL VALUE:

Calories: 300 (approximate)

Fat: 25g (approximate)

Carbohydrates: 15g (approximate)

Fiber: 7g (approximate)

Protein: 2g (approximate)

Sodium: 60mg (approximate)

NOTES

For a richer flavor, add a tablespoon of unsweetened cocoa powder to the avocado mousse mixture.

If the avocado mousse is too thick, add a little more almond milk until you reach the desired consistency.

PREPARATIONS

- In a blender or food processor, combine the avocado flesh, almond milk, lime juice, honey or maple syrup, vanilla extract, and sea salt. Blend until smooth and creamy.
- Divide the avocado mousse between two serving cups or bowls.
- For the Citrus Glaze (Optional): In a small saucepan, combine orange juice, lemon juice, and honey or maple syrup. Heat the glaze gently over low heat until it begins to thicken.
- Drizzle the citrus glaze over the avocado mousse before serving (optional).

NOTES

The citrus glaze is optional, but it adds a refreshing tang to the creamy avocado mousse.

Tropical Fruit Salad with Toasted Nut and Seed Crunch

Portion Size: Serves 2-3 people

PREP TIME: 10 minutes

INGREDIENTS

- 1 cup chopped mango
- 1 cup chopped pineapple
- 1/2 cup chopped kiwi
- 1/2 cup chopped papaya
- 1/4 cup chopped strawberries
- 1/4 cup unsweetened shredded coconut
- 1/4 cup mixed raw nuts and seeds (almonds, pecans, pumpkin seeds)
- 1 tablespoon lime juice
- 1 teaspoon honey (optional)

NUTRITIONAL VALUE:

Calories: 250
Fat: 10g
Carbohydrates: 35g
Fiber: 5g
Protein: 2g
Sodium: 10mg

PREPARATIONS

- In a large bowl, combine the chopped mango, pineapple, kiwi, papaya, and strawberries.
- In a small skillet over medium heat, toast the mixed nuts and seeds for 2-3 minutes, stirring occasionally, until fragrant and slightly browned. Watch them closely to avoid burning.
- Add the toasted nuts and seeds, shredded coconut, and lime juice to the fruit mixture. Toss gently to combine.
- Drizzle with honey, if using, and toss again. Serve immediately.

NOTES

You can substitute other tropical fruits like guava or starfruit for the ones listed in the recipe.

If you don't have a skillet, you can toast the nuts and seeds in a preheated oven at 350°F (175°C) for 5-7 minutes, stirring occasionally.

Feel free to adjust the amount of honey to your taste preference. You can also use other natural sweeteners like stevia or monk fruit.

Decadent Paleo Chocolate Bars

Portion Size: Makes about 8-10 bars   **PREP TIME:** 15 minutes

INGREDIENTS

- 1 cup raw almonds
- 1/2 cup pitted dates
- 1/4 cup unsweetened shredded coconut
- 1/4 cup chopped walnuts or pecans
- 2 tablespoons melted coconut oil
- 2 tablespoons raw cacao powder
- 1/4 teaspoon sea salt
- 1/4 teaspoon ground cinnamon

NUTRITIONAL VALUE

Calories: 250
Fat: 18g
Carbohydrates: 20g
Fiber: 4g
Protein: 4g
Sodium: 30mg

Notes:

You can substitute other nuts or seeds for the chopped walnuts or pecans.

For a richer chocolate flavor, you can use a bit more cacao powder.

These bars can be stored in an airtight container in the refrigerator for up to 2 weeks.

PREPARATIONS

- Pulse the raw almonds in a food processor until they are coarsely crushed. Sometimes you might need to scrape down the sides.
- Add the pitted dates, shredded coconut, chopped walnuts or pecans, melted coconut oil, cacao powder, sea salt, and cinnamon to the food processor. Process until a sticky dough forms.
- Line a small baking dish (around 8x8 inch) with parchment paper. Press the chocolate bar mixture evenly into the prepared baking dish.
- Place in the refrigerator until solid, at least 30 minutes.
- Cut into squares or bars and enjoy!

Refreshing Mint and Melon Sorbet

Portion Size: Makes 4-6 servings   **PREP TIME:** 10 minutes

INGREDIENTS

- 2 cups chopped seedless watermelon (flesh only)
- 1 cup chopped cantaloupe (flesh only)
- 1/4 cup fresh mint leaves
- 1/4 cup water
- 1-2 tablespoons stevia or monk fruit sweetener (to taste)
- 1 tablespoon lime juice

NUTRITIONAL VALUE

Calories: 40

Fat: 0g

Carbohydrates: 10g

Fiber: 1g

Protein: 0g

Sodium: 2mg

Notes:

You can use any type of melon you like for this recipe, such as honeydew or Galia.

If the sorbet becomes too icy after freezing, you can briefly blend it again to achieve a smoother texture.

For a more intense mint flavor, you can add a few drops of peppermint extract instead of fresh mint leaves.

PREPARATIONS

- In a blender, combine chopped watermelon, cantaloupe, mint leaves, and water.
- Blend until smooth and well combined.
- Add stevia or monk fruit sweetener one tablespoon at a time, blending after each addition, until desired sweetness is reached.
- Stir in lime juice.
- Pour the sorbet mixture into a shallow freezer-safe container.
- Freeze until fully frozen, which should take at least 4 hours.
- To serve, let the sorbet soften slightly at room temperature for a few minutes before scooping.

Spiced Pear and Almond Butter Fritters

Portion Size: Makes about 6-8 fritters **PREP TIME:** 15 minutes

INGREDIENTS

- 1 ripe pear, peeled and grated
- 1/4 cup almond flour
- 1/4 cup unsweetened shredded coconut
- 1/4 cup chopped almonds
- 1/4 teaspoon ground cinnamon
- 1/4 teaspoon ground ginger
- 1/8 teaspoon nutmeg (optional)
- 1 tablespoon almond butter
- 1 egg, beaten
- Coconut oil for frying

NUTRITIONAL VALUE

- Calories: 180
- Fat: 10g
- Carbohydrates: 15g
- Fiber: 3g
- Protein: 4g
- Sodium: 30mg

Notes:

You can use other types of nut butter, such as cashew butter or sunflower seed butter (optional, if tolerated), in place of almond butter.

If the batter seems too wet, add a little more almond flour until it reaches a manageable consistency.

Serve these fritters with a drizzle of honey or maple syrup (optional) for an extra touch of sweetness.

PREPARATIONS

- In a medium bowl, combine grated pear, almond flour, shredded coconut, chopped almonds, cinnamon, ginger, nutmeg (optional), and almond butter.
- Mix well until a thick batter forms.
- Mix in the beaten egg after adding it.
- Heat a thin layer of coconut oil in a frying pan over medium heat.
- Using a spoon, scoop portions of the batter into the hot oil, flattening them slightly into fritter shapes.
- Cook for 2 to 3 minutes on each side, or until thoroughly cooked and golden brown. Drain on paper towels to get rid of extra oil.
- Serve warm or at room temperature.

Coconut and Pecan Cookies with a Hint of Cinnamon

Portion Size: Makes about 12-14 cookies

PREP TIME: 10 minutes

INGREDIENTS

1 cup almond flour
1/2 cup unsweetened shredded coconut
1/4 teaspoon baking soda
1/2 teaspoon ground cinnamon
1/4 teaspoon sea salt
1/2 cup unsalted butter, softened
1/2 cup granulated sugar (or a combination of granulated and brown sugar for a richer flavor)
1 large egg
1 teaspoon vanilla extract
1 cup chopped pecans

NUTRITIONAL VALUE

- Calories: 250
- Fat: 14g
- Carbohydrates: 22g
- Fiber: 2g
- Protein: 3g
- Sodium: 60mg

Notes:

You can adjust the amount of cinnamon to your taste preference.

For a chewier cookie, bake for a minute or two less.

If the dough seems too dry, add 1 tablespoon of melted coconut oil or almond milk.

PREPARATIONS

- Preheat oven to 350°F (175°C). Put parchment paper on one side of a baking sheet.
- In a medium bowl, whisk together almond flour, shredded coconut, baking soda, cinnamon, and salt.
- In a separate bowl, cream together softened butter and sugar until light and fluffy. BBlend the egg and vanilla essence until thoroughly blended.
- Mixing until just incorporated, gradually add the dry ingredients to the wet ones.
- Fold in the chopped pecans.
- Drop rounded tablespoons of dough onto the prepared baking sheet, leaving space between cookies for spreading.
- Bake for ten to twelve minutes, until the edges are browned.
- After a few minutes, let the cookies cool on the baking sheet before moving them to a wire rack to finish cooling.

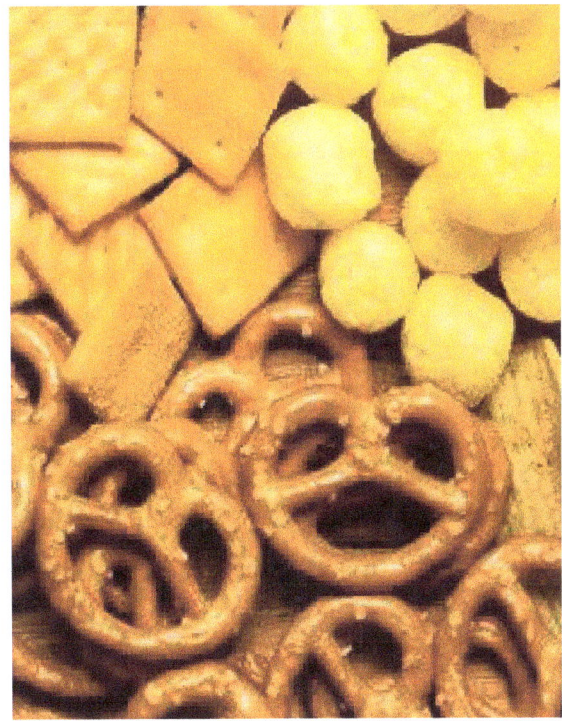

Kid-Friendly Lectin-Free Snack Creations

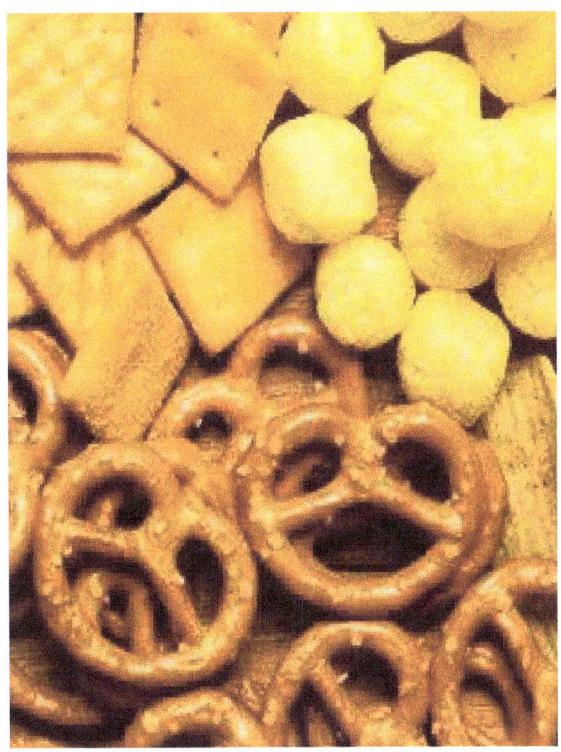

Portion Size: 1 serving

PREP TIME: 5 minutes

INGREDIENTS

- 1/2 cup plain yogurt (optional, if tolerated) or coconut yogurt
- 1/2 cup chopped berries (strawberries, blueberries, raspberries)
- 1 tablespoon unsweetened shredded coconut (optional)
- Stevia or monk fruit sweetener to taste

NUTRITIONAL VALUE

- Calories: 100 (from berries and coconut)
- Fat: 2g (from coconut)
- Carbohydrates: 20g (from berries)
- Fiber: 4g (from berries)
- Protein: 1g (from berries)
- Sodium: 10mg (from berries)

Notes:

You can adjust the amount of stevia or monk fruit sweetener to your taste preference.

For a thicker parfait, use Greek yogurt (optional, if tolerated) or thicker coconut yogurt.

PREPARATIONS

- In a small cup or bowl, spoon in half of the yogurt or coconut yogurt.
- Layer with half of the chopped berries.
- Sprinkle with half of the unsweetened shredded coconut (optional).
- Repeat layers with remaining yogurt or coconut yogurt, berries, and coconut (optional).
- Drizzle with a few drops of stevia or monk fruit sweetener to taste.

Ant on a Log

Portion Size: 4 servings PREP TIME: 5 minutes

INGREDIENTS

- 4 celery sticks, cut into bite-sized pieces
- 2 tablespoons almond butter or cashew butter (optional, if tolerated)
- 1/4 cup raisins or dried cranberries

NUTRITIONAL VALUE

- Calories: 180
- Fat: 8g (from almond butter)
- Carbohydrates: 20g (from celery and raisins)
- Fiber: 4g (from celery and raisins)
- Protein: 4g (from almond butter)
- Sodium: 30mg (from celery and raisins)

PREPARATIONS

- Spread a thin layer of almond butter or cashew butter (optional) on each celery stick.
- Press raisins or dried cranberries into the almond butter or cashew butter (optional) to resemble ants.

Notes:

- If you don't have almond butter or cashew butter, you can use sunflower seed butter (optional, if tolerated).
- You can substitute chopped dried fruits like chopped dates or apricots for the raisins or dried cranberries.

Rainbow Veggie Sticks with Dip

Portion Size: Serves 2-3 people **PREP TIME:** 10 minutes

INGREDIENTS

- For the Vegetables:
- 1 carrot, cut into sticks
- 1 red bell pepper (optional, if tolerated), cut into sticks
- 1 cucumber, cut into sticks
- 1 zucchini, cut into sticks
- For the Dip:
- 1/2 cup coconut yogurt (optional, if tolerated)
- 1 tablespoon chopped fresh herbs (basil, parsley)
- 1 tablespoon lemon juice

Notes:

- You can add other colorful vegetables like broccoli florets or sugar snap peas to create an even more vibrant rainbow effect.
- If you don't have fresh herbs, you can use 1/2 teaspoon dried herbs like basil or parsley instead.
- For a thicker dip, you can add a tablespoon of mashed avocado (optional) to the yogurt or coconut yogurt (optional).

PREPARATIONS

- Wash and chop the vegetables into sticks.
- In a small bowl, combine coconut yogurt (optional, if tolerated), chopped fresh herbs, and lemon juice. Stir until well combined.
- Arrange the veggie sticks on a plate and serve with the prepared dip.

NUTRITIONAL VALUE

- **Calories:** 50 (from vegetables)
- **Fat:** 1g (from vegetables)
- **Carbohydrates:** 10g (from vegetables)
- **Fiber:** 3g (from vegetables)
- **Protein:** 1g (from vegetables)
- **Sodium:** 20mg (from vegetables)

Mini "Pizzas" on Sliced Apples

Portion Size: Makes 4-6 mini pizzas (depending on apple size) **PREP TIME:** 5 minutes

INGREDIENTS

- 2 apples (such as Gala or Honeycrisp)
- 1/4 cup mashed avocado
- 1/4 cup chopped walnuts
- 1/4 cup chopped pecans
- 1/2 teaspoon ground cinnamon

NUTRITIONAL VALUE

- Calories: 150
- Fat: 9g
- Carbohydrates: 18g
- Fiber: 3g
- Protein: 2g
- Sodium: 15mg

NOTES:

You can substitute almond butter (optional, if tolerated) for the mashed avocado for a different flavor profile.

If you don't have walnuts and pecans, you can use other chopped nuts like almonds or cashews (optional, if tolerated).

Drizzle a touch of honey or maple syrup for extra sweetness

PREPARATIONS

- Wash and dry the apples. Slice them horizontally into 1/4-inch thick rounds.
- Spread a thin layer of mashed avocado on each apple slice.
- Sprinkle the chopped walnuts and pecans evenly over the avocado layer.
- Dust each "mini pizza" with a pinch of ground cinnamon.

Sweet & Savory Trail Mix

Portion Size: 1-2 SERVINGS   **PREP TIME:** 5 minutes

INGREDIENTS

- 1/2 cup chopped almonds
- 1/2 cup chopped pecans
- 1/4 cup pumpkin seeds (pepitas)
- 1/4 cup unsweetened dried cranberries
- 1/4 cup chopped apple

NUTRITIONAL VALUE

- Calories: 300
- Fat: 18g
- Carbohydrates: 25g
- Fiber: 5g
- Protein: 6g
- Sodium: 30mg

PREPARATIONS

- In a bowl, combine chopped almonds, pecans, pumpkin seeds, dried cranberries, and chopped apple.
- Toss everything together until well combined.

NOTES:

You can adjust the ingredients to your preference. Add other nuts, seeds, or dried fruits like chopped apricots or raisins (be mindful of added sugars).

For a more "savory" mix, add a sprinkle of ground cinnamon or paprika.

Store the trail mix in an airtight container for up to a week.

Frozen Yogurt Bites

Portion Size: Makes 4-6 frozen yogurt bites **PREP TIME:** 5 minutes

INGREDIENTS

- 1 cup frozen berries (strawberries, blueberries, raspberries)
- 1/2 cup unsweetened almond milk
- 1/4 teaspoon stevia or monk fruit sweetener (optional)

NUTRITIONAL VALUE

Calories: 50

Fat: 2g

Carbohydrates: 8g

Fiber: 1g

Protein: 1g

Sodium: 10mg

PREPARATIONS

- In a blender, combine frozen berries, almond milk, and sweetener (optional). Blend until smooth and pourable.
- Pour the yogurt mixture into silicone molds (ice cube trays can also be used).
- Freeze for at least 3 hours, or until completely solid.

NOTES:

You can use any variety of frozen berries you choose.

For a thicker consistency, add a scoop of chia seeds or flax seeds to the blender.

Let the frozen yogurt bites thaw slightly for a few minutes before enjoying.

Spiced Coconut Crackers

Portion Size:

PREP TIME: minutes

INGREDIENTS

- 1/2 cup almond flour
- 1/4 cup unsweetened shredded coconut
- 1/4 teaspoon sea salt
- 1/4 teaspoon ground cinnamon
- 1/8 teaspoon ground ginger (optional)
- 2 tablespoons melted coconut oil
- 1-2 tablespoons water (optional)

NUTRITIONAL VALUE

- Calories: 40
- Fat: 3g
- Carbohydrates: 3g
- Fiber: 1g
- Protein: 1g
- Sodium: 30mg

PREPARATIONS

- Preheat oven to 350°F (175°C). Put parchment paper on one side of a baking sheet.
- In a medium bowl, whisk together almond flour, shredded coconut, sea salt, cinnamon, and ginger (optional).
- Add the melted coconut oil and thoroughly combine. The mixture should resemble coarse crumbs.
- If the dough seems too dry and doesn't hold together, add water, 1 tablespoon at a time, until a pliable dough forms. Be careful not to overmix.
- Transfer the dough to a lightly floured surface and roll it out thinly, aiming for an even thickness of about 1/8 inch.
- Use a cookie cutter (optional) or a sharp knife to cut the dough into desired shapes.
- Place the crackers on the prepared baking sheet, leaving a little space between them for spreading.
- Bake for 10-12 minutes, or until the edges are golden brown and the crackers are slightly firm to the touch.
- Let the crackers cool completely on the baking sheet before storing or serving.

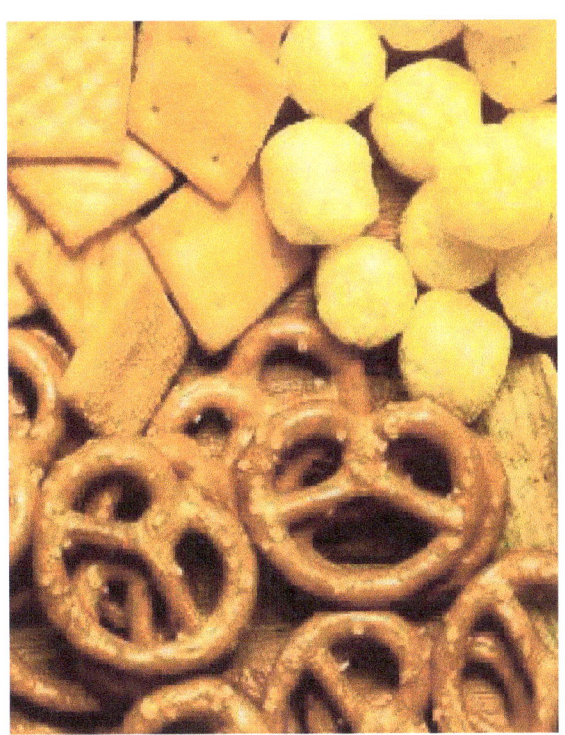

Gluten-Free and Lectin-Free Options

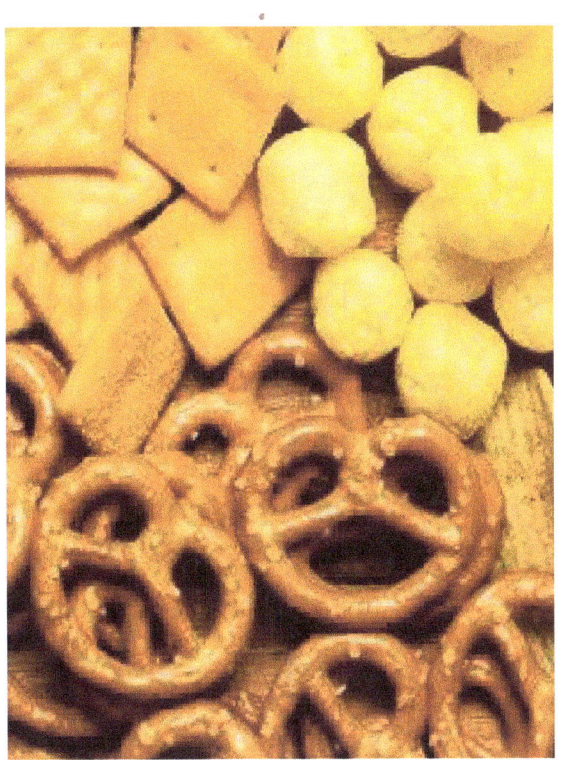

Spicy Shrimp and Veggie Stir-Fry

Portion Size: Serves 2-3 people **PREP TIME:** 10 minutes

INGREDIENTS

- 1 pound medium shrimp (peeled and deveined, optional)
- 1 tablespoon olive oil
- 1 medium zucchini, diced
- 1 cup broccoli florets
- 1 bell pepper (optional, if tolerated), diced
- 1 clove garlic, minced
- 1 tablespoon grated ginger
- 1/4 cup coconut aminos
- 1 tablespoon rice vinegar
- 1 teaspoon cornstarch
- 1/2 teaspoon chili powder (optional)
- 1/4 teaspoon black pepper
- 1 cup cooked cauliflower rice (or regular rice if tolerated)

NUTRITIONAL VALUE

- Calories: 250
- Fat: 10g
- Carbohydrates: 25g
- Fiber: 5g
- Protein: 5g
- Sodium: 400mg (depending on sodium content of coconut aminos)

NOTE:

The sodium content can vary depending on the brand of coconut aminos used.

PREPARATIONS

If using shrimp, pat them dry with paper towels.

In a big wok or skillet, warm up the olive oil over medium-high heat. Add the shrimp (optional) and cook for 2-3 minutes per side, or until pink and opaque. Take out of the pan and place it aside.

Add the diced zucchini, broccoli florets, and bell pepper (optional) to the pan. Stir-fry for 5-7 minutes, or until the vegetables are tender-crisp.

In a small bowl, whisk together coconut aminos, rice vinegar, cornstarch, chili powder (optional), and black pepper.

Transfer the sauce mixture to the veggie pan. Bring to a simmer and cook for 1-2 minutes, or until the sauce thickens slightly.

Add the cooked shrimp (optional) back to the pan and toss to coat in the sauce.

Serve immediately over cooked cauliflower rice (or regular rice if tolerated).

Coconut Curried Chicken Salad

Portion Size: Serves 2-3 people   **PREP TIME:** 10 minutes

INGREDIENTS

- 2 boneless, skinless chicken breasts
- 2 celery stalks, diced
- 1 apple, diced (optional, if tolerated)
- 1/2 cup chopped walnuts
- 1/2 cup unsweetened coconut milk
- 1 tablespoon curry powder
- 1/2 teaspoon turmeric
- 1/4 teaspoon stevia (or to taste)
- 1 tablespoon chopped fresh parsley
- Salt and black pepper to taste
- Lettuce leaves (for serving)

NUTRITIONAL VALUE

- Calories: 400
- Fat: 20g
- Carbohydrates: 15g
- Fiber: 5g
- Protein: 30g
- Sodium: 120mg

NOTE:

The nutritional value can vary depending on the size of the chicken breasts and the brand of coconut milk used.

PREPARATIONS

- Poach the chicken breasts in a pot of simmering water for 15-20 minutes, or until cooked through. Take it out of the saucepan and allow it to cool a little. Shred the chicken with two forks.
- In a large bowl, combine the shredded chicken, diced celery, diced apple (optional), and chopped walnuts.
- In a small bowl, whisk together coconut milk, curry powder, turmeric, stevia, and chopped parsley. To taste, season with salt and pepper.
- Pour the dressing over the chicken salad mixture and toss to coat evenly.
- Arrange a bed of lettuce leaves for serving the chicken salad.

Zucchini Noodle Primavera

Portion Size: Serves 2 people

PREP TIME: minutes

INGREDIENTS

- 2 medium zucchinis
- 1 tablespoon olive oil
- 1 clove garlic, minced
- 8 oz sliced mushrooms
- 1 cup chopped asparagus
- 1/2 cup cherry tomatoes (optional, if tolerated)
- 1/4 cup chopped fresh parsley
- 1 tablespoon lemon juice
- 1/2 teaspoon paprika
- Salt and black pepper to taste

NUTRITIONAL VALUE

- Calories: 180
- Fat: 8g
- Carbohydrates: 15g
- Fiber: 4g
- Protein: 2g
- Sodium: 150mg

NOTES:

- You can add other vegetables to this recipe, such as chopped bell peppers or shredded carrots.
- For a spicier dish, add a pinch of red pepper flakes to the dressing.
- If you don't have fresh parsley, you can substitute 1 teaspoon of dried parsley.

PREPARATIONS

- Spiralize the zucchinis to make zucchini noodles with a spiralizer.
- Over medium heat, warm up the olive oil in a big skillet. Once fragrant, sauté the minced garlic for 30 seconds.
- Add the sliced mushrooms and asparagus to the skillet and cook for 5-7 minutes, or until softened and slightly browned.
- If using cherry tomatoes, add them to the pan with the vegetables and cook for an additional 2-3 minutes, until they soften slightly.
- Add the zucchini noodles to the pan and toss with the cooked vegetables.
- In a small bowl, whisk together lemon juice, olive oil, paprika, salt, and black pepper.
- Pour the dressing over the zucchini noodle mixture and toss to coat evenly.
- Cook for an additional 1-2 minutes, or until the zucchini noodles are heated through.
- Take off the heat and add the freshly cut parsley.
- Serve immediately.

Almond Flour Pancakes

Portion Size: Makes about 4 small pancakes   **PREP TIME: 20** minutes

INGREDIENTS

- 1/2 cup almond flour
- 2 large eggs
- 1/3 cup unsweetened almond milk
- 1/4 teaspoon ground cinnamon
- 1/4 teaspoon baking powder
- 1/8 teaspoon sea salt
- 1 tablespoon melted coconut oil (for greasing the pan)
- Optional toppings: fresh berries, maple syrup (optional, if tolerated)

NUTRITIONAL VALUE

- Calories: 120
- Fat: 8g
- Carbohydrates: 5g
- Fiber: 2g
- Protein: 4g
- Sodium: 60mg

Notes:

- You can adjust the amount of cinnamon or add a pinch of nutmeg for additional flavor.
- If the batter seems too thick, add a tablespoon or two of additional almond milk.
- For a thicker pancake, use 1/3 cup of batter per pancake

PREPARATIONS

- In a medium bowl, whisk together almond flour, baking powder, cinnamon, and sea salt.
- In a separate bowl, whisk together the eggs and almond milk until well combined.
- After adding the wet ingredients to the dry ingredients, whisk to mix them just enough. A few little lumps are acceptable.
- Set a skillet that has been gently oiled over medium heat. In the pan, melt one teaspoon of coconut oil.
- Each pancake should have 1/4 cup of batter added to the heated griddle.
- Cook for 2 to 3 minutes on each side, or until well cooked and golden brown.
- Continue with the remaining batter, spritzing the pan with extra coconut oil as needed.
- Serve pancakes immediately with your favorite toppings.

Baked Salmon with Herb Crust (Gluten-Free & Lectin-Free)

Portion Size: **PREP TIME:** minutes

INGREDIENTS

- 1 (6-ounce) salmon fillet, skin-on or skinless
- 1/4 cup almond flour
- 2 tablespoons melted coconut oil
- 1 tablespoon chopped fresh parsley
- 1 tablespoon chopped fresh dill
- 1/2 teaspoon dried thyme
- 1/4 teaspoon sea salt
- 1/4 teaspoon black pepper

NUTRITIONAL VALUE

- Calories: 450
- Fat: 30g
- Carbohydrates: 5g
- Fiber: 2g
- Protein: 40g
- Sodium: 450mg

NOTES:

You can substitute other fresh herbs like basil or rosemary for parsley and dill.

If you don't have almond flour, you can use another type of nut flour like cashew flour or pecan flour.

PREPARATIONS

- Preheat oven to 400°F (200°C). Line a baking sheet with parchment paper.
- Pat the salmon fillet dry with paper towels. Sprinkle salt and pepper on the salmon's two sides.
- In a small bowl, combine almond flour, melted coconut oil, chopped parsley, dill, thyme, salt, and pepper. To make a crumbly mixture, thoroughly combine.
- Place the salmon on the prepared baking sheet. Spread the herb crust mixture evenly over the top of the salmon, pressing gently to adhere.
- Bake the salmon for 15-20 minutes, or until the flesh is opaque and flakes easily with a fork.

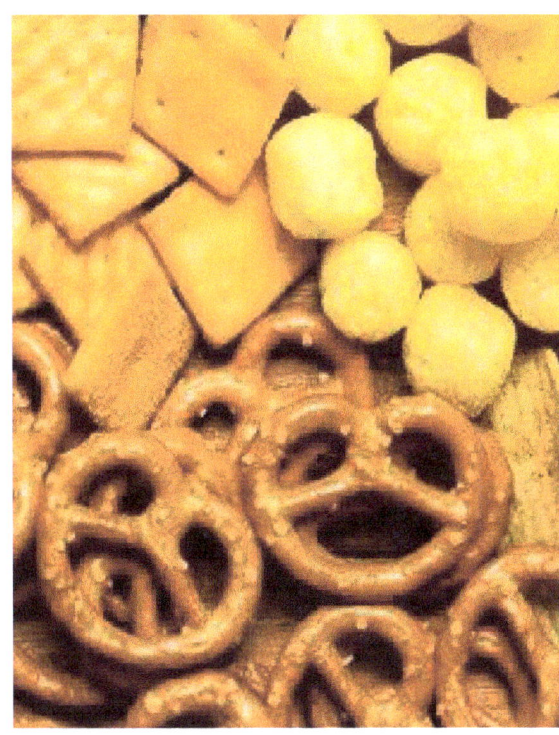

Dairy-Free and Lectin-Free Substitutions

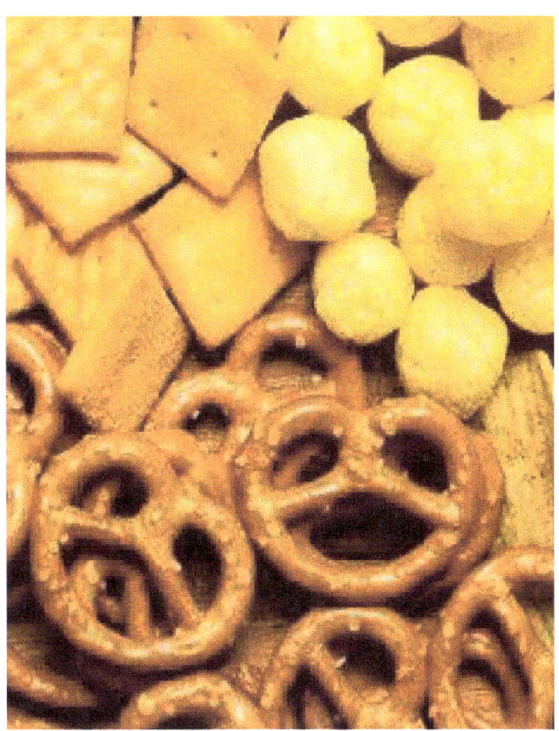

Creamy Avocado Pasta Sauce

Portion Size: : Makes enough sauce for 2-3 servings   **PREP TIME:** 10 minutes

INGREDIENTS

- 2 ripe avocados, pitted and halved
- 1/2 cup chopped fresh basil
- 1/4 cup freshly squeezed lemon juice
- 1 tablespoon olive oil
- 1 clove garlic, minced
- 1/4 teaspoon sea salt
- 1/4 teaspoon black pepper
- 1/4 cup reserved pasta water (optional)
- Cooked gluten-free pasta of choice (amount depends on serving size)

NUTRITIONAL VALUE

- Calories: 220
- Fat: 18g
- Carbohydrates: 10g
- Fiber: 5g
- Protein: 2g
- Sodium: 180mg

NOTES:

You can add a pinch of red pepper flakes for a touch of spice.

For a richer flavor, add a tablespoon of nutritional yeast (optional) to the blender with other ingredients.

Leftover sauce can be stored in an airtight container in the refrigerator for up to 1 day. However, the color may darken slightly due to avocado oxidation.

PREPARATIONS

- Cook your chosen gluten-free pasta according to package instructions. Reserve about 1/4 cup of the pasta water before draining.
- In a blender or food processor, combine the avocado flesh, chopped basil, lemon juice, olive oil, garlic, salt, and pepper.
- Blend until smooth and creamy. If the sauce is too thick, add a tablespoon or two of the reserved pasta water to achieve desired consistency.
- Coat the cooked spaghetti thoroughly by tossing it in the creamy avocado sauce.
- Serve immediately and enjoy!

Coconut Yogurt Parfait

Portion Size: 1 SERVING **PREP TIME:** 5 minutes

INGREDIENTS

- 1 cup unsweetened coconut yogurt (alternative for dairy yogurt)
- 1/2 cup chopped berries (strawberries, blueberries, raspberries)
- 1/4 cup unsweetened shredded coconut
- To taste, add stevia or monk fruit sweetener (optional).
- Fresh mint leaves for garnish (optional)

NUTRITIONAL VALUE

- Calories: 200
- Fat: 14g
- Carbohydrates: 18g
- Fiber: 3g
- Protein: 4g
- Sodium: 30mg

NOTES:

- Any kind of berry will work just well.
- Feel free to substitute the shredded coconut with chopped nuts or granola (be mindful of lectins in granola).
- For a thicker consistency, you can freeze the coconut yogurt for a few hours before layering the parfait.

PREPARATIONS

- In a small serving glass or bowl, layer half of the coconut yogurt.
- Top with half of the chopped berries.
- Sprinkle with half of the unsweetened shredded coconut.
- Repeat layers with remaining yogurt, berries, and coconut.
- Drizzle with a touch of stevia or monk fruit sweetener, if desired.
- Garnish with a fresh mint leaf (optional) and serve.

Cauliflower Rice Soup

Portion Size: Serves 4-6 people   **PREP TIME:** 10 minutes

INGREDIENTS

- 1 head cauliflower, riced (or 1 bag pre-riced cauliflower)
- 4 cups vegetable broth
- 1 tablespoon olive oil
- 1 medium onion, chopped
- 2 cloves garlic, minced
- 1/2 teaspoon turmeric
- 1/2 teaspoon cumin
- Salt and black pepper to taste
- 1 cup unsweetened coconut milk (full-fat for creamier soup)
- 1/4 cup chopped fresh parsley (optional)

NUTRITIONAL VALUE

- Calories: 150
- Fat: 8g
- Carbohydrates: 15g
- Fiber: 4g
- Protein: 4g
- Sodium: 400mg (depending on broth used)

NOTES:

- You can add other vegetables to this soup, such as chopped carrots, celery, or broccoli.
- For a richer flavor, you can substitute chicken broth for the vegetable broth (optional, if tolerated).

PREPARATIONS

- Warm up the olive oil in a big pot over medium heat. Add the chopped onion and simmer for about 5 minutes, or until softened.
- Stir continuously for an additional minute after adding the minced garlic.
- Stir in the riced cauliflower, turmeric, and cumin. Cook for 2-3 minutes, until fragrant.
- After adding the veggie broth, bring it to a boil. Reduce heat and simmer for 10-15 minutes, or until the cauliflower is tender.
- Using an immersion blender or a regular blender in batches, puree the soup until smooth and creamy. If desired, you can add extra broth to change the consistency.
- Stir in the coconut milk and season with salt and black pepper to taste. Heat through for another minute.
- Serve hot, garnished with chopped fresh parsley (optional).

Avocado Toast with Poached Eggs

Portion Size: Serves 1 person **PREP TIME:** 10 minutes

INGREDIENTS

- 2 slices whole-wheat or gluten-free bread (toasted)
- 1 ripe avocado, sliced
- 2 large eggs
- 1 tablespoon white vinegar
- Salt and black pepper to taste
- Optional toppings: Everything bagel seasoning, hot sauce, lemon juice

NUTRITIONAL VALUE

- Calories: 350
- Fat: 18g
- Carbohydrates: 25g
- Fiber: 7g
- Protein: 12g
- Sodium: 200mg (depending on bread used)

NOTES:

- For a vegan option, use mashed chickpeas instead of the poached egg.
- You can adjust the amount of vinegar and cooking time for the poached eggs to your desired level of doneness.
- Leftover avocado toast can be stored in an airtight container in the refrigerator for up to 1 hour

PREPARATIONS

- Add roughly two inches of water to a small saucepan. Bring the water to a simmer (gentle bubbles). Add the vinegar.
- Crack each egg into a small separate bowl.
- Once the water is simmering, gently swirl the water with a spoon to create a vortex. Carefully slide each egg into the center of the vortex.
- Cook the eggs for 3-4 minutes, or until the whites are set and the yolks are runny.
- While the eggs are cooking, toast the bread slices.
- Toast the bread and then spread the avocado slices on it.
- Using a slotted spoon, remove the poached eggs from the water and place them on top of the avocado toast.
- To taste, add salt and black pepper for seasoning.
- Add your favorite toppings, such as everything bagel seasoning, hot sauce, or a squeeze of lemon juice (optional).

Tropical Smoothie Bowl

Portion Size: 1 SERVING   **PREP TIME:** 10 minutes

INGREDIENTS

- 1 cup frozen mango chunks
- 1 cup frozen pineapple chunks
- 1/2 cup unsweetened almond milk
- 1/4 cup chopped banana (optional, if tolerated)
- 1 tablespoon chia seeds
- 1/2 teaspoon ground ginger (optional)
- 1/4 teaspoon stevia or monk fruit sweetener (optional)
- For Toppings (choose your favorites):

- Fresh berries (strawberries, blueberries, raspberries)
- Sliced kiwi
- Chopped mango or pineapple
- Unsweetened shredded coconut
- Chopped nuts or seeds (almonds, pumpkin seeds)
- Hemp seeds (optional)

NUTRITIONAL VALUE

- Calories: 250
- Fat: 4g
- Carbohydrates: 40g
- Fiber: 5g
- Protein: 2g
- Sodium: 10mg

NOTES:

- Feel free to adjust the sweetness level to your preference by adding more or less stevia or monk fruit sweetener

PREPARATIONS

- In a high-speed blender, combine frozen mango chunks, frozen pineapple chunks, unsweetened almond milk, chopped banana (optional), chia seeds, ground ginger (optional), and stevia or monk fruit sweetener (optional).
- Blend until smooth and creamy. You may need to stop the blender a couple of times to scrape down the sides and ensure everything is evenly blended.
- Pour the smoothie mixture into a bowl.
- Add your desired toppings. Get creative and personalize your bowl with a variety of colorful and flavorful options!

Vegan and Lectin-Free Recipes for Plant-Based Enthusiasts

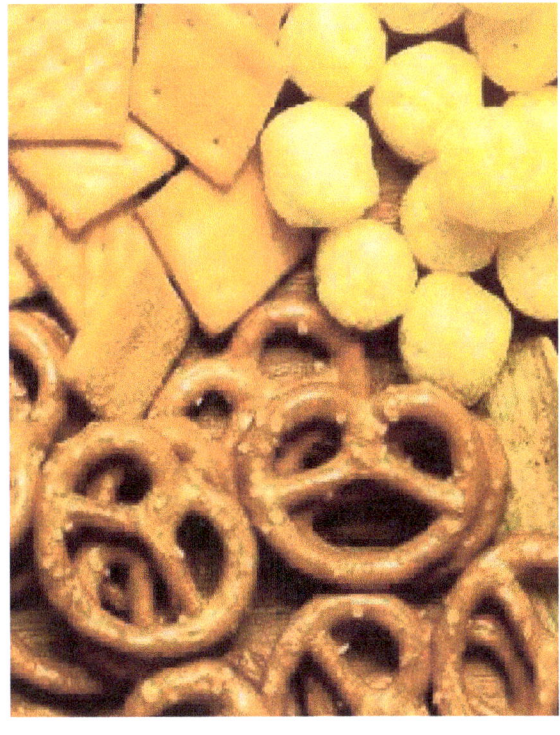
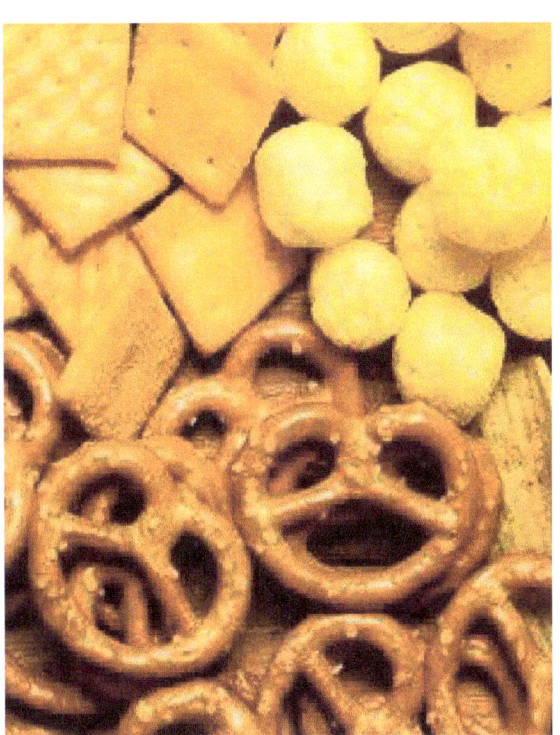

Lentil Soup with Vegetables

Portion Size: Serves 4-6 people   **PREP TIME:** 10 minutes

INGREDIENTS

- 1 cup dry green lentils
- 4 cups vegetable broth
- 2 carrots, chopped
- 2 celery stalks, chopped
- 1 onion, chopped
- 2 cloves garlic, minced
- 4 cups chopped kale or spinach
- 1 tablespoon olive oil
- 1 teaspoon ground cumin
- 1/2 teaspoon turmeric
- 1/2 teaspoon sea salt
- 1/4 teaspoon black pepper
- Fresh herbs (optional): chopped parsley, cilantro

NUTRITIONAL VALUE

Calories: 250
Fat: 5g
Carbohydrates: 40g
Fiber: 15g
Protein: 15g
Sodium: 350mg

PREPARATIONS

- Rinse the lentils in a fine-mesh strainer.
- Warm up the olive oil in a big pot over medium heat. Add the chopped onion and simmer for about 5 minutes, or until softened.
- Add the chopped carrots and celery to the pot and cook for another 5 minutes, stirring occasionally.
- Add the garlic, cumin, turmeric, salt, and pepper to the pot. Stir for a minute to release the fragrance of the spices.
- Pour in the vegetable broth and rinsed lentils. After bringing to a boil, lower the heat and simmer the lentils for 20 to 25 minutes, or until they become soft.
- Stir in the chopped kale or spinach and cook for an additional 2-3 minutes, or until wilted.
- Taste and adjust seasonings as needed.
- Serve hot, garnished with fresh chopped herbs (optional).

Black Bean Burgers

Portion Size: Makes 4 burgers **PREP TIME:** 15 minutes

INGREDIENTS

- One can (15 oz) of rinsed and drained black beans
- 1 cup cooked quinoa
- 1/2 cup chopped red onion
- 1/4 cup chopped bell pepper (optional)
- 1/4 cup chopped fresh cilantro
- 1 tablespoon ground flaxseed
- 3 tablespoons water
- 1 teaspoon chili powder (optional)
- 1/2 teaspoon cumin
- 1/2 teaspoon smoked paprika
- 1/4 teaspoon sea salt
- 1/4 teaspoon black pepper
- Cooking spray or avocado oil

NUTRITIONAL VALUE

- Calories: 300
- Fat: 10g
- Carbohydrates: 40g
- Fiber: 10g
- Protein: 15g
- Sodium: 250mg

PREPARATIONS

- In a large bowl, mash together the drained black beans with a fork until slightly chunky.
- Add the cooked quinoa, chopped red onion, chopped bell pepper (optional), chopped cilantro, flaxseed meal, water, chili powder (optional), cumin, paprika, salt, and pepper.
- Mix well to combine all ingredients. If the mixture seems too wet, add a little more flaxseed meal or breadcrumbs (optional).
- Form the mixture into 4 equal patties.
- Heat a skillet with cooking spray or avocado oil over medium heat.
- Add the burger patties to the skillet and cook for 4-5 minutes per side, or until golden brown and heated through.
- Serve on hamburger buns with your favorite toppings like lettuce, tomato (optional, if tolerated), avocado, and vegan mayo (optional).

Tofu Scramble

Portion Size: Serves 2 people

PREP TIME: 10 minutes

INGREDIENTS

- One 14-oz block of firm tofu that has been drained and pressed
- 1 tablespoon olive oil
- 1/2 onion, diced
- 1/2 bell pepper (optional, if tolerated), diced
- 1/4 teaspoon turmeric
- 1/4 teaspoon paprika
- 1/4 teaspoon black pepper
- 1/4 cup chopped fresh vegetables (spinach, mushrooms, etc.) - optional
- 1/4 cup chopped fresh herbs (parsley, cilantro)
- 2 tablespoons soy sauce (optional)
- 1/4 cup water

NUTRITIONAL VALUE

- Calories: 250
- Fat: 12g
- Carbohydrates: 10g
- Fiber: 2g
- Protein: 20g
- Sodium: 320mg (depending on soy sauce usage)

NOTES:

You can experiment with different vegetables in your tofu scramble. Chopped mushrooms, spinach, tomatoes (optional, if tolerated), or broccoli florets work well.

For a spicier scramble, add a pinch of red pepper flakes while cooking.

PREPARATIONS

Drain and press the tofu block to remove excess moisture. Wrap the tofu in a clean kitchen towel and place a heavy object (like a cutting board or a pot) on top for at least 15 minutes.

While the tofu presses, heat olive oil in a large skillet over medium heat. Add diced onion and bell pepper (optional) and cook until softened, about 5 minutes.

Break apart the compressed tofu with a fork or your hands. Add the crumbled tofu to the pan with the vegetables.

Sprinkle the tofu with turmeric, paprika, and black pepper. Stir to coat evenly.

Add chopped fresh vegetables (optional) and cook for a few minutes until softened.

Pour in the water and soy sauce (optional). Cook for another 5 minutes, or until the tofu is heated through and slightly browned.

Stir in chopped fresh herbs and cook for another minute.

Serve immediately with toast, avocado slices, or your favorite breakfast sides.

Roasted Chickpea Salad with Herbs

Portion Size: Serves 2 people

PREP TIME: 10 minutes

INGREDIENTS

- One can (15 oz) of rinsed and drained chickpeas
- 1 tablespoon olive oil
- 1/2 teaspoon paprika
- 1/4 teaspoon cumin
- 1/4 teaspoon sea salt
- 1/4 cup chopped cucumber
- 1/4 cup chopped tomatoes (optional, if tolerated)
- 1/4 cup chopped fresh herbs (mint, parsley)
- 2 tablespoons lemon juice
- 1 tablespoon olive oil (for dressing)

NUTRITIONAL VALUE

- Calories: 220
- Fat: 8g
- Carbohydrates: 20g
- Fiber: 5g
- Protein: 10g
- Sodium: 180mg

Notes:

- You can add other chopped vegetables to this salad, such as chopped bell peppers (optional, if tolerated) or chopped red onion.
- For a creamier texture, mash a few of the chickpeas before adding them to the salad.
- You can eat this salad cold or warm.

PREPARATIONS

- Preheat oven to 400°F (200°C). Line a baking sheet with parchment paper.
- Pat the chickpeas dry with a clean kitchen towel.
- In a medium bowl, toss the chickpeas with olive oil, paprika, cumin, and sea salt.
- Spread the seasoned chickpeas on the prepared baking sheet in a single layer.
- Roast the chickpeas for 20-25 minutes, or until crispy and golden brown.
- While the chickpeas roast, prepare the salad dressing. Olive oil and lemon juice should be combined in a small basin.
- In a serving bowl, combine the roasted chickpeas, chopped cucumber, tomatoes (optional, if tolerated), and chopped fresh herbs.
- Pour the lemon-olive oil dressing over the salad and toss to coat evenly.
- Serve right away or store in the fridge for up to three days.

Vegan Lectin-Free Coconut Curry with Vegetables

Portion Size: 2 SERVES

PREP TIME: 10 minutes

INGREDIENTS

1 tablespoon coconut oil
1 medium onion, chopped
2 cloves garlic, minced
1 tablespoon curry powder
1 teaspoon ground turmeric
1/2 teaspoon ground ginger (optional)
1 (14-ounce) can full-fat coconut milk
1 cup vegetable broth
1 cup chopped broccoli florets
1 cup chopped cauliflower florets
1/2 cup chopped bell pepper (optional, if tolerated)
1/2 cup chopped zucchini
1/4 cup chopped fresh cilantro
1 tablespoon chopped fresh parsley
Sea salt and black pepper to taste
Cooked brown rice or quinoa (for serving)

NUTRITIONAL VALUE

- Calories: 400 (approximate, may vary depending on rice/quinoa)
- Fat: 25g
- Carbohydrates: 35g
- Fiber: 8g
- Protein: 10g
- Sodium: 150mg (may vary depending on added salt)

Notes:

Feel free to adjust the amount of curry powder for your desired level of spice.

To add a touch of sweetness, you can stir in a teaspoon of stevia or monk fruit sweetener after adding the vegetables.

PREPARATIONS

- In a big pot or Dutch oven, warm the coconut oil over medium heat. Add the chopped onion and simmer for about 5 minutes, or until softened.
- Add minced garlic and cook for an additional minute, stirring constantly, until fragrant.
- Stir in curry powder, turmeric, and ginger (optional). Cook for another minute, allowing the spices to release their aroma.
- Pour in the coconut milk and vegetable broth. Bring to a simmer.
- Add chopped broccoli, cauliflower, bell pepper (optional), and zucchini. Reduce heat and simmer for 10-12 minutes, or until the vegetables are tender-crisp.
- Stir in chopped fresh cilantro and parsley. Add sea salt and black pepper according to taste.
- Serve hot over cooked brown rice or quinoa.

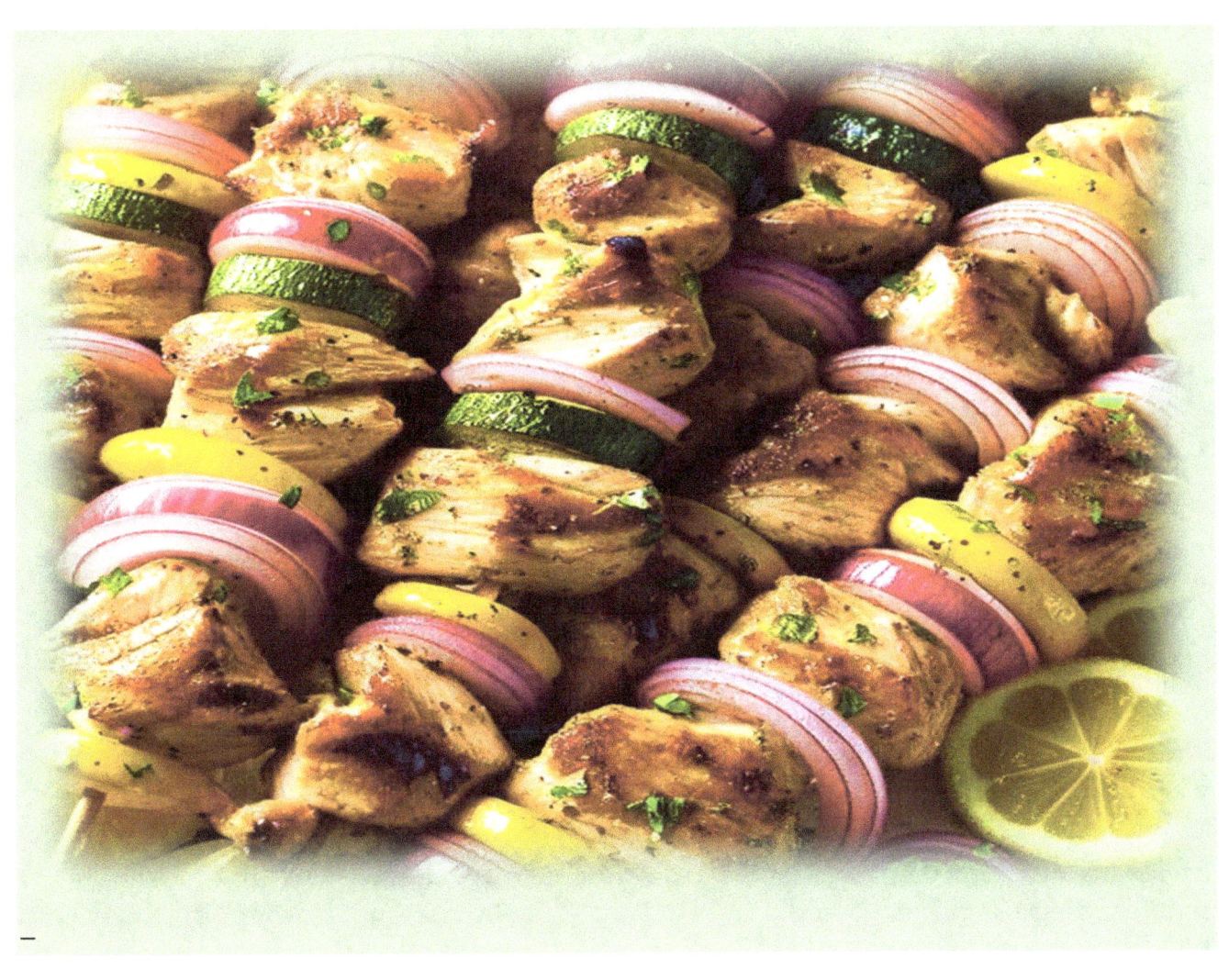

Conclusion

Embracing a Healthier You: A Lectin-Free Snacking Journey

As you reach the end of this journey into the world of lectin-free eating, a world brimming with vibrant flavors and nourishing options, we can confidently say this: a healthier you awaits. By incorporating lectin-free snacks into your daily routine, you've taken a significant step towards a more vibrant and energized life.

Making Lectin-Free Snacking a Habit:

Imagine reaching for a satisfying and healthy snack throughout your day. Here are some tips to seamlessly integrate lectin-free snacks into your routine:

Plan Your Snacks: Dedicate a few minutes each week to plan your lectin-free snacks. Prepare chopped vegetables in advance, portion out nuts and seeds, or freeze some delicious yogurt parfaits for a grab-and-go option.

Prep is Key: Invest in reusable containers to portion out snacks and keep them readily available in the refrigerator or pantry. This makes healthy choices the easy choice when hunger strikes.

Snack Throughout the Day: Don't wait until you're ravenous! Regular snacking helps regulate blood sugar levels and prevents overeating later. Aim for two to three between-meal snacks each day.

Get Creative!: This book is just the beginning. Explore the vast world of lectin-free recipes and experiment with different flavors and textures.

Beyond Snacks: A Holistic Approach to Wellness

Remember, lectin-free snacks are just one piece of the puzzle. Embracing a healthier lifestyle is an ongoing journey, and delicious choices pave the way for lasting change. Here are some more methods to think about:

Prioritize Whole Foods: Build your meals around whole, unprocessed foods like fruits, vegetables, healthy fats, and lean proteins.

Stay Hydrated: Water is essential for optimal health. Aim for eight glasses of water per day to keep your body functioning at its best.

Move Your Body: Engaging in regular physical activity is essential to general health. Find an activity you enjoy, whether it's brisk walking, dancing, or yoga, and make it a part of your routine.

Embrace Sleep: Adequate sleep is vital for physical and mental health. Every night, try to get 7–8 hours of good sleep.

By incorporating these habits alongside your lectin-free snacks, you're well on your way to promoting a healthy gut, boosting energy levels, and ultimately, feeling your best.

Remember, this journey is about progress, not perfection. Celebrate your successes, learn from your challenges, and most importantly, enjoy the delicious and nourishing path towards a healthier you.

www.ingramcontent.com/pod-product-compliance
Lightning Source LLC
Chambersburg PA
CBHW062116220526
45471CB00010B/3758